W9-BDL-536

A Diet for All Seasons

A Diet
for All Seasons

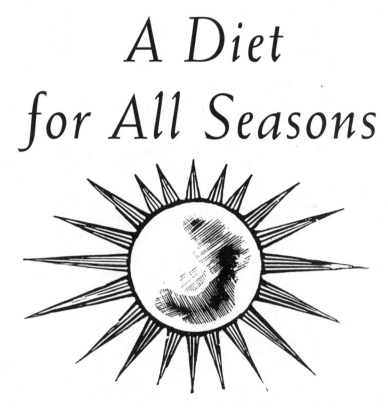

ELSON M. HAAS, M.D.
with Eleonora Manzolini

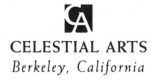

CELESTIAL ARTS
Berkeley, California

Copyright © 1995 by Elson M. Haas, M.D. All rights reserved. No part of this book may be reproduced in any form, except for brief review, without permission of the publisher. For further information, you may write to:

CA Celestial Arts Publishing
P.O. Box 7123
Berkeley, California 94707

Cover and text design by Toni Tajima

Excerpt from *Tropic Cooking* by Joyce LeFray Young, copyright © 1987 by Joyce LeFray Young. Reprinted by permission of Ten Speed Press, Berkeley, CA.

Excerpts from *The Tao of Cooking* by Sally Pasley, copyright © 1982 by Sally Pasley. Reprinted by permission of Ten Speed Press, Berkeley, CA.

Excerpts from *The Airola Diet and Cookbook* by Paavo Airola, copyright © 1981 by Paavo Airola. Reprinted by permission of Health Plus Publishers.

Excerpts from *The Book of Whole Meals: A Seasonal Guide to Assembling Balanced Vegetarian Breakfasts, Lunches and Dinners* by Annemarie Colbin, copyright © 1985 by Annemarie Colbin. Reprinted by permission of Ballantine Books.

Excerpts from *Still Life With Menu (Revised)* by Mollie Katzen, copyright © 1988, 1995 by Mollie Katzen. Reprinted by permission of Ten Speed Press, Berkeley, CA.

Excerpts from *The New Laurel's Kitchen* by Laurel Robertson, Carol Flinders, and Brian Rupenthal, copyright © 1976 by The Blue Mountain Center of Mediation, Inc. Reprinted by permission of Ten Speed Press, Berkeley, CA.

Excerpts from *The Enchanted Broccoli Forest (Revised)* by Mollie Katzen, copyright © 1982, 1995 by Mollie Katzen. Reprinted by permission of Ten Speed Press, Berkeley, CA.

Excerpts from *Eat Well, Be Well Cookbook* by Metropolitan Life Insurance Company, copyright © 1986 by Metropolitan Life Insurance Company, Chefs Staff. Reprinted by permission of Simon & Schuster Publishing.

Excerpts from *Stress, Diet, and Your Heart* by Dean Ornish, M.D., copyright © 1982 by Dean Ornish, M.D. Reprinted by permission of Henry Holt and Co.

Excerpts from *Fast Vegetarian Feasts (Revised)* by Martha Rose Shulman, copyright © 1986 by Martha Rose Shulman. Reprinted by permission of Doubleday Books.

Excerpt from *The Self-Healing Cookbook*, by Kristina Turner, copyright © 1987 by Kristina Turner. Reprinted by permission of Earthtones Press.

Excerpts from *Cosmic Cookery* by Kathryn Hannaford, copyright © 1974 by Kathryn Hannaford. Reprinted by permission of the author.

Excerpt from *Fit for Life* by Marilyn and Harvey Diamond, copyright © 1985 by Marilyn and Harvey Diamond. Reprinted by permission of Warner Books.

Excerpts from *Moosewood Cookbook (Revised)* by Mollie Katzen, copyright © 1977, 1992 by Mollie Katzen. Reprinted by permission of Ten Speed Press, Berkeley, CA.

Excerpt from *Dr. Braly's Food Allergy and Nutrition Revolution* by James Braly, M.D., copyright © James Braly and Laura Torbert. Reprinted by permission of the author. Available from Kaets Publishing.

Excerpts from *Hippocrates Diet and Health Program*, copyright © 1984 by Ann Wigmore. Reprinted by permission of Avery Publishing Group. 800-548-5757

Library of Congress Cataloging-in-Publication Data

Haas, Elson M., 1947-
    A diet for all seasons / Elson M. Haas.
        p.   cm.
    ISBN 0-89087-732-7
    1. Cookery (Natural foods) 2. Nutrition I. Manzolini, Eleonora. II. Title.
TX741.H33 1995
641.5'63—dc20
                                             94–39129
                                                CIP

Printed in the United States

First Printing, 1995

1 2 3 4 5 — 99 98 97 96 95

CONTENTS

RECIPE TABLE OF CONTENTS . . . . *vii*

PREFACE . . . . *xi*

INTRODUCTION 1

PART I: BUILDING BLOCKS FOR SEASONAL NUTRITION

CHAPTER 1: GUIDELINES FOR A HEALTHY DIET 7

   Food Groups—Old and New 8

   Ten Key Components of a Healthy Diet 10

   A Review of Recommended Dietary Changes 22

CHAPTER 2: YOUR IDEAL DIET 25

   Individual Needs 27

   Changing Your Diet 30

   Daily Schedule 32

   Supplements to the Diet 35

CHAPTER 3: BASICS FOR THE IDEAL DIET 39

   Kitchen Basics 39

   A Few Tips and Shortcuts 44

   For Those Who Wish to Avoid Fats 45

   About Storing 46

CHAPTER 4: RECIPES FOR ALL SEASONS 47

   Some Basic Recipes 48

   Wheat-Free Recipes 64

   Milk/Egg-Free Recipes 66

   Butter-Free Spreads 71

   Quinoa Recipes 73

   Special Snacks for Kids (And Their Folks) 76

PART II: SEASONAL MENU PLANS AND RECIPES 83

CHAPTER 5: SPRING 87

CHAPTER 6: SUMMER 113

CHAPTER 7: AUTUMN 141

CHAPTER 8: WINTER 173

PART III: SPECIAL DIETS, DETOXIFICATION,
AND OTHER HEALTH GUIDELINES 207

CHAPTER 9: SPECIAL DIETS 211

   Fat-Free Diet 211

   Natural Hygiene/Raw Foods Diet 216

   Macrobiotic Diet 220

   Ayurveda Diet 225

CHAPTER 10: DETOXIFICATION AND REJUVENATION 231

CHAPTER 11: OTHER HEALTH GUIDELINES 237

RECIPE BOOK BIBLIOGRAPHY 243

INDEX 245

RECURSE TABLE OF CONTENTS

RECIPE TABLE OF CONTENTS

▼ FOR ALL SEASONS ▼

Dr. Sun's Granola 48

General Salad Ingredients 49

Mixed Sprout Salad 50

Cold Rice Salad Variation 51

Low-Fat, Low-Salt Vinaigrette 52

Joe Terry's Miso Magic Dressing 53

Vegetable Broth 54

Thick (Spicy) Vegetable Soup 55

Salsa 56

Guacamole 56

Tostadas 57

Steamed Veggie Platter 58

Sesame Salt (Gomasio) 58

Rainbow Rice 59

Chop Suey 60

Homemade Ketchup 61

Tomato Sauce 62

Quick Spicy Tomato Sauce 63

Wheat-Free Pie Crust 64

The Universal Cracker Recipe 65

Tofu Sour Cream 66

Tofu Mayonnaises 67

Rejuvelac 68

Seed Cheese 69

Seed Yogurt 69

Bean Spreads (or Dip) 70

Sweet Carrot Butter 71

Sesame-Squash Butter 72

Mexican Quinoa with Spinach 73

Colorful Quinoa Salad with
    Raspberry Yogurt Dressing 74

Raspberry Yogurt Dressing 74

Victoria's Quinoa Cake with Lemon Sauce 75

Lemon Sauce 75

Frozen Juice Pops 76

Dr. Elson's Nice Cream 77

Yogurt Freezes 77

Nut Milks 78

Halvah 79

Fruit Bars 80

Puffed Rice Balls 80

Almond Cookies 81

Tofu-Nut Spread 81

✤ SPRING ✤

Pasta with Garbanzos 90

Avocado Dressing 90

Puréed Carrot Soup 91

Tofunaise 91

Tomato-Caper Sauce 92

Miso-Tahini Dressing 92

Vegetable Minestrone 93

Pesto Sauce 94

Couscous Salad 95

Polenta 96

Tomato-Lentil Sauce 96

Watercress Bisque 97

Sweet and Sour Tempeh or Tofu 98

Sweet and Sour Sauce 98

Strawberry-Rhubarb Pudding 99

White Bean Florentine Soup 100

Artichoke Stew 101

Fettuccine Primavera with Curry 102

Brown Rice with Peas and Fava Beans 103

Zucchini Flowers with Tofu Filling 104

Lime-Garlic Shrimp 105

Green Jade Soup 106

Watercress Salad 107

Pollution Solution Dressing 108

Rice and Vegetable Salad 109

Creamy Parsley Dressing 109

Pasta with Greens and Feta 110

✿ SUMMER ✿

Breakfast Rice 116

Stuffed Bell Peppers 117

Crêpes with Fruit 118

Scrambled Tofu 119

Chicken "en Chemise" 120

Fruit Sorbet 121

Fruit Kanten (Jelled Fruit Dessert) 121

Moussaka 122

Honey-Mustard Vinaigrette 122

Corn Bread 123

Peanut-Apple Butter 123

Mexican Salad Bowl 124

Baked Dill Salmon 125

Salad of Belgian Endive 125

Tofu Aspic 126

Ratatouille 127

Swiss Chard Stuffed with Barley 128

Dr. Haas' Spicy Coleslaw 129

Fresh Corn and Tomato Soup 130

Russian Beet Salad 131

Israeli Salad 132

Tao Salad 133

Tao Dressing 133

Zucchini with Garlic and Tomatoes 134

Rice Crust Pizza 135

Couscous Casserole 136

Pasta with Marinated Vegetables 137

Banana-Yogurt Freeze 138

Sunshine Bars 139

∾ AUTUMN ∾

Fillet of Sole Florentine 144

Lasagna 145

Prune and Apricot Compote 146

Avo-Miso-Tofu Topping 146

Walnut-Miso Sauce 147

Carob-Tofu Mousse 147

Millet Breakfast Cake with Orange Sauce 148

Orange Sauce 148

Mushroom Turkey Breast 149

Wilted Spinach Salad 150

Millet Croquettes 150

Brazilian Feijoada 151

Grilled Swordfish with Pineapple Mustard 152

Warm Red Cabbage Salad 153

Pasta alla Boscaiola 154

Pears in Black Cherry Juice 155

Simple Potato and Tomato Casserole 156

Chicken and Tomatillos 157

Reduced-Fat Parsley Mashed Potatoes 158

Sea Bass with Seasonal Pepper Coulis 159

Dr. Haas' Split Pea Soup 160

Kasha Cream with Sunflower Seeds 161

Garlic Soup 162

Thai Garlic Soup 163

Veggie Burgers 164

Confetti Quinoa 165

Tempeh Cacciatore 166

Rich Jalapeño Corn Bread 167

Szechuan-Style Sweet and
    Sour Chinese Cabbage 168

Carrot Bread 169

Carrot Hash Browns 170

Shrimp Creole 171

❄ WINTER ❄

Cracked Wheat with Raisins and Walnuts 176

Cream of Broccoli Soup 176

Roasted Turkey 177

Mushroom Sauce 177

Stir-Fried Vegetables with Tempeh or Tofu 178

Oatmeal Spice Cookies 179

Curried Chicken Breast 180

Millet, Squash, and Adzuki Bean Stew 181

Apple-Raisin Compote 181

Snapper Parmentiere 182

Arame Carrots, Scallions, and Corn 183

Lentil Soup with Barley and Dulse 184

Pumpkin Pie.................................185

Butternut Bisque 186

Norimaki Sushi 187

Rice-Lentil Loaf with Green Sauce 188

Green Sauce 189

Onion Soup 190

Leeks and Cauliflower with Bechamel 191

Macaroni and Tofu Au Gratin....................192

Stuffed Baked Apples.........................193

Russian Soup.................................194

Russian Cabbage Borscht 195

Hot and Sour Soup...........................196

Hot and Sour Dressing 197

Kasha with Mushrooms, Water Chestnuts,
    and Celery 198

Cabbage Leaves Stuffed with Kasha,
    with Creamy Tofu Sauce....................199

Vegetarian Chili.............................200

Spicy Nut Sauce 201

Basmati Rice 'n' Eggs 202

Soya-Carob-Nut Brownies 203

Carob Icing.................................203

Tofu-Banana Cream Pie........................204

❧ SPECIAL DIETS ❧

FAT-FREE

White Bean and Pesto Purée.........................212

Tomato Vinaigrette.............................213

Couscous Flan 214

Parsley-Mint Sauce.............................214

Creamy Garlic Sauce...........................215

Bread Pudding 215

NATURAL HYGIENE/RAW FOODS

Sweet Corn Gazpacho...........................217

Raw Hummus.................................218

Sauerkraut.................................218

Raw Apple Pie...............................219

MACROBIOTIC

Mushroom Miso Soup 222

Brown Rice and Adzuki Beans
    with Arame 223

Bok Choy in Ginger Sauce 224

Apple Mousse.................................224

AYURVEDA

Dahl Soup 227

Vegetable Curry 228

Cucumber Raita...............................229

Date and Orange Chutney 229

PREFACE

With the overwhelmingly positive response to *Staying Healthy with Nutrition,* Eleonora Manzolini and I were inspired to write a more "hands-on" version for readers interested primarily in the meal plans and delicious recipes found in the book. Many people have purchased *Staying Healthy with Nutrition* for its thorough nutritional information. Obviously we believe in the importance of that information, but we also understand the need for accessibility. People want to reach to their cookbook shelves for immediate nutritional guidance and recipes which they trust will make a difference in their diet and health. Here, in *A Diet for All Seasons,* we have distilled the valuable information of the previous book with a clear emphasis on meal plans and wonderful recipes for healthy, seasonal living.

Eleonora and I have put our energies together again to invent more wonderful cuisine creations for you and those close to you. *A Diet for All Seasons* includes new recipes for each season and chapters on special topics with recipes to enhance the new information. We feel that *A Diet for All Seasons* will give you an eating plan for maintaining optimum health throughout the year.

We're sure that you'll enjoy the book's simple yet savory recipes. We're equally certain that you will feel better and better the longer you choose to eat this way. When I was a child, my father, Martin, had a wonderful way of getting me to eat my vegetables. He'd say, "Kid, if you eat that for a hundred years, you'll live a long time." And you know, I still have that carrot in my pocket!

Be Well,

Elson M. Haas, M.D.

"For the Earth is the Lord's, and the fullness thereof"

Romans 10:26

INTRODUCTION

Let me make one thing perfectly clear—*A Diet for All Seasons* is not a fad diet book. It is an eating plan for the entire year and an extremely simple, "ideal" approach for longevity of health and vitality. I do not want you to "go on a diet" (diets generally don't work); I want you to change your eating habits and make positive choices to create the result you wish to achieve. Remember, your body and health are by-products of the way you live and the food choices you make. A focus on the eating plan and recipes in this book will allow you to clear adverse habits and create a healthy eating program.

The Seasonal Diet is just that; it makes use of fresh, seasonal foods that are eaten mainly around the time of year they are naturally harvested. This allows the most vitality and the least amount of chemical treatment for bug protection and storage. *A Diet for All Seasons* is also primarily vegetarian, but is flexible to include some fish and poultry recipes if you choose to add these to your diet, as I occasionally do. Furthermore, your Ideal Diet avoids the overuse of common food allergens and congestors like cow's milk products, wheat, refined flour products, and refined sugars.

For some of you, *A Diet for All Seasons* will require some dramatic changes; for others, simple shifts and fine tuning may be all you need. Changing habits may also take a little work on the emotional level, as often your desire for a particular food or food flavor serve to satisfy some displaced emotional need. If you feel you require emotional support to change your habits, I encourage you to seek it. However, if you can rely on your own motivation and willpower to work toward your goal, just go for it!

Along with a **positive attitude toward life, management of stress, and maintenance of a regular exercise regimen,** this **dietary approach** will support your continuous creation of health. Complete health and vitality are difficult to achieve without these important contibutions.

I have read and reviewed hundreds of diet and nutrition books in the last twenty years of my nutritional study and practice, and I have not found as sound an approach to healthy eating as we present in this book. Our diet is good for you and it is good for our planet.

You will find that following the suggestions in *A Diet for All Seasons* will:

* Improve your energy
* Reduce (or optimize) your weight
* Clear existing allergies
* Help prevent chronic disease
* Add quality to your years
* Align you closer to nature and its rhythms
* Help you attune to other healthful aspects of life

Evaluate your health now, and then follow this plan for the year. At the end of that time, assess your health again to determine just how well you are doing. If you want a very in-depth and accurate assessment tool, you may utilize the Health Bank Account from the Questionnaire in *Staying Healthy with Nutrition*. The many patients of mine who have made the transition from their diets to our seasonally-based natural diet—and cleared their personal addictions—give me great reports. If your experience is anything like theirs, you will find yourself dancing more easily through life, healthier in body and mind.

There is no longer any doubt that **food and diet influence health and disease**, although the conventional medical establishment is slow to emphasize such findings. If you truly desire a change in your body and state of health, you can do this all or at least in part by changing your diet and lifestyle habits. And with individual lifestyle changes comes collective health improvement. Once you take more responsibility for your own health, the cost savings for our health care system will be phenomenal.

In my experience, the benefit of making lifestyle changes has far greater use and service than "quick fix" medical attempts at treating disease. I have never been entirely fulfilled by the formulaic approach I learned in medical school: name a disease, prescribe a treatment, and make sure the patient doesn't get worse or experience adverse side effects. A bit of nutritional counseling really only takes a few minutes out of an office visit and could greatly affect a person's life.

The prospect of a transformational experience arising from my visit with a patient is what continues to impassion me about medical/health practice. I do not feel that I have done my job until my patients discover tools and gain insights for positively altering the course of their lives.

So, let's begin with a few bits of advice for healthy and happy eating:

- ◆ Your ideal meal should be about the size of your two cupped hands. If you are still hungry, take another small portion.
- ◆ Eat your main meal at lunch.
- ◆ Chew your food very well; relax and breathe between mouthfuls.
- ◆ Eat quietly, sitting at a table. Do not watch TV, read the newspaper, or listen to loud music.
- ◆ Do not drink ice cold beverages with meals. Preferably do not drink with meals at all. It is best to drink before a meal.
- ◆ Sit quietly for five minutes after finishing your meal.

In this book, you will be guided to eat a nature-based, nurture-filled diet oriented to the "new four" food groups—fruits, vegetables, whole grains, and protein-containing foods. This is a low-fat, high-vitality eating plan. It also orients you toward eating certain types of food at certain times of the day for optimum digestion and health. Many medical problems begin in the intestinal tract; therefore, good health also begins there. We do not encourage much eating after nightfall; if anything, take only a light snack. Drink lots of good quality water throughout the day, but not with your meals: thirty minutes before or an hour after meals is best. And make new statements to yourself, such as: "I do not need nearly as much food to support my energy and health. It matters what I eat; everything I consume becomes part of me. I do not need to snack between meals. I am drinking plenty of good water. I enjoy exercising daily to make me healthy and vital," and anything else that affirms the inherent knowledge that you can create optimum health in your body, mind, and heart.

Our recipes have been hand-selected and tested by Eleonora and her cooking students. They are simple to prepare, healthful, and very tasty; we know you will enjoy them.

I encourage you to seek health and healing in every level of your life. I have, and I can tell you it's worth it. Now, in my forties, I must stay healthy to keep up with my work and my two young children. I exercise regularly and work in the garden. I keep my stress low and my attitude high. And, of course, I continue to pay close attention to my nutritional habits.

I am excited to present you with a guide for feeling wonderful. Enjoy *A Diet for All Seasons*. Let it nourish you, your family, and your friends with good health and good food.

PART I

BUILDING

BLOCKS

FOR

SEASONAL

NUTRITION

"Happiness: A good bank account, a good cook, and a good digestion."

JEAN-JACQUES ROUSSEAU

CHAPTER 1

GUIDELINES FOR A HEALTHY DIET

A healthful diet involves many components. Nutrition has gotten very complex, with a continual flood of new information—both insightful truth and propaganda—surfacing daily in the news and various publications. Yet nutrition can be simple. We believe this book provides the key information to keep healthy eating simple and accessible to the body—easy to digest, assimilate, and utilize. Basically, we need to return to our instincts for proper nutrition.

Our natural locale provides the best and most wholesome foods av`ilable to us. Local stores, however, display a continuing array of fancy new packages, boxes, and cans hyped by equally flashy advertising. Profitability is the key motivation in the food industry, and much of what we are buying is packaging and advertising, which often costs more than the actual food in the product. If we took some of this big business money and paid all mothers (and fathers and brothers) to grow food and prepare wholesome, natural meals, we would take a big step toward the health and well-being of ourselves and our planet. Though this would be revolutionary if done on a mass level, it is exactly what we need to do individually—go back to the basics and redevelop our nutrition. To do this, we need to change our thinking and the conditioning of an entire century of advertising that has so strongly influenced and molded the diets of Americans, and, really, the diets of people worldwide. To begin with, let us first look at one of the earlier misconceptions still taught in most schools of our nation: "four-food-group" nutrition.

FOOD GROUPS—OLD AND NEW

This complex, important concept regarding the basics of our diet is a challenging area of nutrition. For nearly a century, mainstream nutritional thought has centered on the "basic four" food groups: meats, dairy products, cereal grains, and fruits and vegetables. But many of us feel that this approach is archaic, unhealthy, and part of the reason for the large increase in chronic degenerative diseases in recent years.

There are several reasons why the "basic four" approach is difficult to change. The main reason is that people have been conditioned to believe that these categories of foods are equally important, and that meats, as well as milk, butter, and eggs, are crucial parts of a good meal. This belief is taught in school and exemplified in the cafeteria diet. All of these foods, of course, can be consumed and are nutritionally helpful—but only in modest amounts, not as two out of four of the main food groups as is recommended. Even younger children need far less of these high-protein, high-fat foods than we think, even though these foods do stimulate growth. Protein deficiency is highly unlikely in a balanced diet, as are most mineral and vitamin deficits, and we need less protein to maintain health than most people assume.

The food industry is very resistant to changing the "basic four." Billions have been spent in creating and advertising products that are less healthy for us than the basic foods that nature provides. And many high-fat, high-salt, and high-sugar foods are so intensely promoted that our profit-oriented industry often has more influence on our diet and health than do informed parents and nutritionists. We are convinced by advertising to try these new boxes, cans, and frozen treats that imitate our natural wholesome foods and create refuse for the Earth and for our bodies. Thus, this concept of the "basic four," created by the power of the dairy, meat, and breakfast cereal industries—and supported by the medical kingdom and educational system—leaves the farmer with only one category to cover all the nourishing fruits and vegetables.

Finding the proper balance of these foods is our first important step in creating a healthy diet. A starch-centered diet has been the native or traditional diet throughout the world during the last ten centuries. This means our main foods were complex carbohydrates high in fiber and nutrients and low in calories. It is the fat in our foods that contributes the most calories. The simple sugars and refined sugars also add up.

This starch-centered diet, as I said, has been the typical native diet. Which carbohydrate is used, however, varies with the culture. Traditional Asian cultures used mainly rice, with some wheat; the East Indian diet was similar, with more wheat; in the Middle East, the staple was wheat; Europeans ate wheat and potatoes; and the

Native Americans used a large amount of corn. These cultures also used some peas or beans to balance the grains and make complete proteins, and many local vegetables were added. This main diet was usually supplemented with smaller amounts of seasonal fruits, milk products, and animal foods.

As technology developed and humans moved up the ladder of success, richer living meant richer foods. Meats, eggs, cheeses, and milk became associated with success. No longer did we need to hunt and move with the seasons. We could pen animals and milk or slaughter them for food. With more technology, shelf life replaced health life. A rejection of the "peasant" diet went hand in hand with this high-fat diet. The refinement of foods was also part of this move "up." As I have discussed, these factors have not improved nutrition. In fact, they have been steps backward in terms of nutritional health. What we need is a "new basic four" food groups.

Our new basics start with ten food groups, the foods nature provides—fruits, vegetables, whole grains, legumes, nuts, seeds, dairy products and eggs, fish, fowl, and red meats.

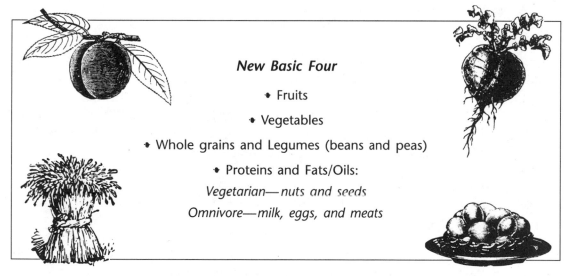

New Basic Four

- Fruits
- Vegetables
- Whole grains and Legumes (beans and peas)
- Proteins and Fats/Oils:

Vegetarian—nuts and seeds

Omnivore—milk, eggs, and meats

The main thrust is the de-emphasis on the meats and dairy products, which need to be combined into one category. The vegetables and the whole grains and legumes are the most significant groups and should be the largest part of the diet.

The specific individual proportions of these groups vary somewhat from person to person and season to season, as we will discuss more fully later. Let us now look at the different components that, I believe, we should bring together to make up our new, healthy diet.

TEN KEY COMPONENTS OF
A HEALTHY DIET

• Natural foods	• Tasty and appealing foods
• Seasonal foods	• Variety and rotation
• Fresh foods	• Food combining
• Nutritious foods	• Moderation
• Clean foods	• Balance

These are not necessarily listed in order of importance. A balanced diet and moderate consumption of foods, without regular overeating, are likely the most important components of a healthy diet, especially on a long-term basis. Other aspects, such as food combining or rotating foods, may be more important in the fine-tuning of our diet or in the treatment of special problems, such as poor digestion or food allergies. However, following these ten guidelines preventively will assure us of keeping our bodies, especially our digestive systems and immune systems, functioning at optimum capacity.

Some of these "components" may also overlap. Freshness and nutritiousness or seasonality and variety may often include the same characteristics and choices in foods.

Which foods are tasty and appealing is a more personal thing—to some this may mean a beautiful, colorful salad and to others a burger and fries. This has a lot to do with the conditioning of our taste buds and brains, which may be the most difficult aspects to change in order to create a healthier diet.

❧ NATURAL FOODS ❧

It is my belief and experience that natural foods are best. The closer our foods are to the garden, fields, and orchards, the more energy, vitality, and nutrients we will obtain per calorie of food consumed. Many packages contain chemicals or metals that pose toxicity concerns; in addition, the packaging itself is often a costly waste product that may not be recyclable, and thus, creates digestive problems for the Earth.

Fruits, nuts, seeds, vegetables, whole grains, and legumes should constitute the majority of our diet, at least 80–90 percent. People eating much more than 10–15 percent of their diet in the form of animal foods should reevaluate their choices, as the high-fat and low-fiber content of these foods can be detrimental to health in the long run.

❧ Seasonal Foods ❧ (Indigenous Diet)

Eating seasonally—choosing foods that are available and grown in our own area—keeps us attuned to the Earth, its elements, and the cycles of nature. It gets us thinking about gardens and being able to pick our own food. Seasonal eating is also the most economical dietary pattern and gives us potentially the cleanest foods, as less chemicals are needed to store or ship them.

My first book, *Staying Healthy With the Seasons*, focused on nutrition through the seasons, with many concepts and practical suggestions about seasonal awareness and diet. Since seasonal eating is also the focus of this book, I want to describe what this term means.

Throughout the year, our environment provides us with the best foods to protect us from the climates, support our health, and keep us in balance. For example, in summer's hottest months, the juiciest of fruits are available. Fruits and fruit juices help to cool the body. In contrast, in cold and wet winter, foods that require more cooking are the most prevalent. Before the advent of technology, these were foods that stored well and were protected by shells or hard skins. They are the grains, nuts, and seeds, and the hard squashes, tubers, and root vegetables—foods that are higher in protein and fats. Be aware that food availability may vary somewhat around the normal harvest time, even by a couple of months, due to weather differences, crop timing, and refrigeration.

Being aware of and using the foods as they are available will help reattune us to nature and, most importantly, to the cycles of our bodies. This is an essential step in attaining and maintaining health. More advice on seasonal nutrition can be found later in this book.

❧ Fresh Foods ❧

Eating fresh foods is one of the healthiest aspects of a diet. Fresh foods include, obviously, foods from nature—fruits, vegetables, grains, nuts, beans, and seeds. Most milk and animal products are included. Fruits and vegetables are best eaten as fresh as possible, but most of these foods store well for several weeks. Whole grains and legumes generally keep for years after harvesting. Nuts and seeds must be more carefully stored (closed containers in a cool, dark place, or refrigerated), as they may easily go rancid because of their oil content. Rancidity causes the biggest problems, however, in milk and animal products: spoilage can cause microbial diseases, since bacteria, viruses, and parasites grow very well in these substances.

As previously noted, eating seasonally allows us to get the freshest produce. Fresh eating means getting as close to the garden, field, or orchard as possible: eating an apple or apricot off a tree, gathering a salad from the garden, or cooking some "just-picked" sweet corn.

❧ Nutritious Foods ❧

Eating a nutritious diet primarily means acquiring all the vitamins, minerals, amino acids, and fatty acids that our bodies need to function optimally. It also means eating specific foods that contain optimum levels of many nutrients. The fresher the foods, the higher they are in potential nutrients. Industrial processing of foods greatly diminishes the level of nourishment.

When I speak of a nutritious diet, I am referring to the focus throughout this book—the consumption of a high percentage of whole foods, as fresh as possible. Eating a variety of foods also allows a greater balance of nutrients. Many processed and refined foods are enriched or fortified to make them more "nutritious." This helps some, but is a distant second to the nourishment received from natural, fresh foods.

❧ Clean Foods ❧

The term "clean diet" refers to two important areas. The first regards consuming chemical-free foods as much as possible. Specifically, this means avoiding chemical additives and chemically treated foods, as well as foods containing refined sugar and flour. Finding organically grown produce and organic (untreated) poultry, beef, and eggs is becoming even more important as pollution worsens in our world. Buying organic foods grown by farmers and ranchers will let them know there is a market that will support them, as opposed to the unconscionable, high-chemical-using producers.

"Clean" also means washing and storing food properly to avoid spoilage and contamination. Washing fresh produce with water and even soap or diluted Clorox bleach (which can remove more germs) before eating or cooking is helpful to clean off the dirt, bugs, or chemicals. Packing food properly for storage in plastic bags or containers will protect it longer as well. Keeping ourselves and our homes, kitchen counters, and utensils clean also protects us and others from spreading disease. Drinking clean, filtered, chemical-free water is also very important.

❧ TASTY AND APPEALING FOODS ❧

Eating a diet that is tasty and appealing satisfies our senses. The more we make each meal a feast for our eyes and mouths, the more it nourishes the deeper levels of our being. It is necessary that our diets be gratifying, and if we do not eat foods we enjoy, we will not be completely satisfied. Color and visual appeal are as important as taste, because they improve `ppetite and enjoyment of the foods. Often, the food tastes especially good when someone has taken the time to prepare a beautiful meal.

All foods have characteristic flavors. Our attraction to some of these flavors, and thus to certain foods, is inherent in our natures, while other tastes are learned or conditioned. To make positive changes in our diet, we need to work at changing our tastes, or, really, developing new tastes. A lot of unnatural or concentrated sweet and salty flavors in foods, as well as chemical tastes, have taken people away from simple, natural eating. To return to or support the many components of the healthy diet discussed here, we may need to recondition ourselves to enjoy the true natural flavors of the real foods of the Earth.

❧ VARIETY AND ROTATION ❧

Eating a variety of foods provides us with a variety of nutrients, thus preventing any marked deficiencies. That is, of course, if the variety of foods we choose is mainly nutritious. If we vary pizza, franks, and hamburgers from day to day, our diet is not going to be very balanced. Eating and varying many of the whole foods will assure a proper amount of nutrients without excesses of potentially harmful levels of sugars, fats, or even protein.

Rotating our diet means eating different foods from day to day and not repeating the same foods every day. This reduces potential food allergies, which can result from repeatedly stimulating our body's immune and cellular systems with the same nutritional biochemistry. Common foods that may generate allergies include cow's milk, wheat, eggs, soybeans, peanuts, corn, beef, coffee, chocolate, tomatoes, yeast, shellfish, and mushrooms.

We may also be genetically sensitive or allergic to foods, or we may have developed allergies through other stresses or illnesses we have experienced. If we do not feel well after we eat—with fatigue, irritability, or specific symptoms such as nasal congestion, itching, or skin rashes—we might want to find out what foods may be responisble. We may then wish to eliminate those foods for a while and go on a very specific four-day rotation diet, with any specific food consumed on one day not again consumed in the next three following days, thereby allowing our body to deal with it and clear it completely, reducing the constant stimulation to our immune system that can occur when we consume a food daily.

❧ FOOD COMBINING ❧

Food combining allows us to better digest and optimally utilize the foods and their inherent nutrients. Many people overstress their digestive tracts by eating a large number of foods at each meal. Our culture has been conditioned more to the balanced meal than to the balanced diet, and people may eat foods from all the different groups at each sitting. This is very taxing on the body, and may in part be why, in America, there is so much digestive disease from stomach to colon. Simple meals of a few ingredients each, using a variety of foods over time, with concern about balancing our diet over the day or week, is a more healthful overall approach to eating.

The basic principles of food combining are as follows:

1. *Fruits are eaten by themselves or with other fruits.* Fruits are high-water-content, simple-sugar foods. They digest very easily and may move through our digestive tract rapidly. When eaten with other foods, they tend to remain and ferment in the stomach. The only exception is that citrus fruit and nuts seem to be handled well together, possibly because the citric acid assists in the digestion of the nuts. A combination of fruit (simple carbohydrate) and cereal grain (complex carbohydrate) is tolerated well by most people. Oatmeal with a sliced banana, apple, or raisins, for example, makes a healthy and delicious meal.

2. *Proteins and starches are not eaten together.* Basic proteins such as meats, poultry, fish, eggs, and milk products require maximum stomach acid levels for best digestion, mainly because of their higher fat content. Nuts and seeds are also better digested with good hydrochloric acid production. Starches, or complex carbohydrates, are digested best in a relatively more alkaline stomach. These foods include whole grains, pastas, potatoes, and breads. When proteins and starches are combined, their stimulation to the digestive juices generates a conflicting response and creates a medium that digests neither food very well. This may lead to indigestion, gas, bloating, abdominal discomfort, and a poor utilization of nutrients.

3. *Combine protein and vegetables or starch and vegetables.* Following the first two rules leaves meals that focus on vegetables with either a protein or starch

complement. Some legumes may be combined with the starch, particularly whole grains, to provide all the essential amino acids. These meals allow the body to best digest the foods and utilize their nutrients. This is a difficult change to make, as it conflicts with our ingrained nutritional concepts and many of the meals that people commonly eat, such as meat and potatoes, fish and pasta, cheese or lunch meat sandwiches, pizza, and even the basic hamburger or hotdog on a bun. So, food combining can be a major undertaking, though a positive one for many people. It aids digestion of meals and keeps excess weight off.

4. *Do not eat more than one protein per meal.* Mixing more than one protein, such as eggs and ham or cheese and meat, can be a little taxing on the digestive tract and often provides an excessive amount of fat and protein.

Food combining is especially important for any of us who have sensitive digestive tracts or intestinal problems. I believe it also helps prevent wearing out our digestive organs too early. Many people consider food combining an extreme that is too difficult to carry out. However, if we do not try it out to see how we feel, we will never know.

❧ MODERATION ❧

Eating moderately, not overeating or undereating, is the basic first habit of good nutrition. Many nutritionists feel that overeating, especially on a regular basis, is the worst thing we can do to our body. The term "overeating" applies to not only the total amount of food consumed but also, as we will see in the next section, to the overconsumption of specific foods leading to improper dietary balance. Overconsumption or abuse of sugars, fats, protein, salt, and chemicals can lead to disastrous results. We must be careful to control the intake of foods that contain large amounts of these ingredients.

Eating too much food at any time, as most of us have experienced, causes great stress on the body. After a meal, much more blood is sent to our digestive organs, and we are often sedated and unable to move very well until digestion is completed many hours later. Regular overeating also tends to reduce our exercise potential, and this, along with increased calorie intake, contributes to weight increase. Almost all obesity, other than from hormonal imbalance, is caused by overconsumption of calories along with physical underactivity. Obesity leads to increased susceptibility to most of the serious and chronic diseases, such as hypertension, heart disease, diabetes, and cancer.

❧ BALANCE ❧

Eating a balanced diet is important to maintaining long-term health. However, the concept of a balanced diet is one of the most controversial topics in the nutritional field. Very few authorities agree on the specifics of this balance, though there seems to be general agreement on the trends. In this section, I will discuss the following five aspects of balance:

- **Macronutrients**—proteins, fats, and carbohydrates.
- **Micronutrients**—vitamins, minerals, amino acids, and fatty acids.
- **Food groups**—fruits, vegetables, grains, legumes, nuts, seeds, dairy products, eggs, fish, poultry, and meats.
- **Flavors**—sour, bitter, sweet, spicy, and salty, and **Colors**—red, orange, yellow, green, blue, purple.
- **Acid-alkaline**—acid-forming and alkalizing foods.

❧ *Balance—Macronutrients*

How much of each of the carbohydrates, fats, and proteins we need will be discussed further in upcoming sections. (Chapters 2–4 in *Staying Healthy with Nutrition* discuss the three macronutrients in detail.) Here I review specifically the basics of these important nutrients and give my suggestions for the right balance. Carbohydrates, which include simple sugars and starches, provide our bodies and cells with easily usable energy. Proteins provide active biochemicals and amino acids, the building blocks of body tissues. Fats provide lubrication and protection, as well as fuel for our bodies. An excess or deficiency of any of the macronutrients can generate problems, so the art of nutrition is to create a diet with the right balance.

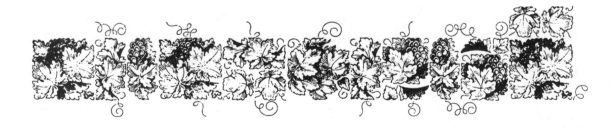

FOOD SOURCES OF THE MACRONUTRIENTS

PROTEINS	FATS		CARBOHYDRATES		
	Saturated	*Unsaturated*	*Complex*	*Simple*	*Refined*
eggs	coconut oil	vegetable oils	grains	fruit	pastry
milk	palm oil	mayonnaise	legumes	honey	refined flour
cheese	animal fat	nuts	hard squash	malt syrup	bread (white)
nuts	butter	seeds	whole grains	maple syrup	cookies
seeds	mayonnaise		breads	molasses	donuts
legumes	whole milk		pasta	other	candy
fish	cheese			natural	soft drinks
poultry	eggs			sweeteners	sugar
meats	meats				
	lard				
	bacon				

MACRONUTRIENTS IN THE DIET—OLD BALANCE AND NEW GOALS

	Average American Diet	*New Goals**
Carbohydrates	46%	60%
	22% complex	45% complex
	6% natural sugars	10% natural sugars
	18% refined sugars	5% refined sugars
Protein	12%	15%
Fat	42%	25%
	7% polyunsaturated	8% polyunsaturated
	19% monosaturated	10% monounsaturated
	16% saturated	7% saturated

*may range from 60–70% carbohydrates, 10–20% protein, 20–30% fat

❖ *Balance—Micronutrients*

There are about 53 essential nutrients—those substances that our body needs in order to carry out its many functions, but that it does not make, at least in sufficient amounts to provide for our needs. In other words, essential nutrients are substances that we need to obtain from food or additional supplements. These include the vitamins and minerals as well as the essential amino acids from protein foods and the essential fatty acids from oils.

To obtain all of these nutrients, we need to eat a variety of natural, fresh, tasty, and nutritious foods. Still, in this day and age, with the diminishing nutrients in the soil and the high amount of food processing, it is not easy to obtain all of our nutrients from food. That is why I often suggest a general supplement for those who are not eating a completely balanced and wholesome diet or who have any signs or symptoms of a possible deficiency. Many people choose to take a general vitamin-mineral supplement and even additional amino acid formulas or essential fatty acids as insurance that they are obtaining all of these needed nutrients.

ESSENTIAL NUTRIENTS

Amino Acids	Vitamins	Minerals
Isoleucine	A—retinol and carotene	Calcium
Leucine	B_1—thiamine	Chloride
Lysine	B_2—riboflavin	Chromium
Methionine	B_3—niacin	Cobalt
Phenylalanine	B_5—pantothenic acid	Copper
Threonine	B_6—pyridoxine	Fluoride
Tryptophan	B_{12}—cobalamin	Iodine
Valine	Biotin	Iron
Arginine**	C—ascorbic acid	Lithium*
Histidine**	Choline	Magnesium
	D—calciferol	Manganese
Fatty Acids	E—tocopherol	Molybdenum
	Folic acid	Nickel*
Linoleic acid	Inositol	Phosphorus
Linolenic acid	K—quinones	Potassium
	P—bioflavonoids	Rubidium*
	PABA—para-aminobenzoic acid	Selenium
		Silicon
		Sodium
		Strontium*
		Sulfur
		Tin*
		Vanadium
		Zinc

*may not be essential

**these are "semiessential," needed in special times of growth and development

✤ *Balance—Food Groups*

"Food groups" is a very broad term that can mean many different things, such as the basic food groups discussed earlier in this chapter or specific classifications of foods, such as the cruciferous vegetables (broccoli, cauliflower, Brussels sprouts, and cabbage). We use the term here to refer to the larger categories of food, such as fruits, vegetables, grains, and legumes. We need to obtain a proper balance among these foods to support the other components of this healthy diet.

As I mentioned, our ideal food group balance will not be the same all year round; even the proportions of the different macronutrients will vary with the seasons. But the following list provides good general guidelines, ranking the groups from those we should consume most to those we should eat least.

FOOD GROUP PRIORITIES: OMNIVOROUS		
1. Vegetables	6. Poultry, organic	11. Fish, freshwater
2. Whole grains	7. Seeds	12. Poultry, nonorganic
3. Fruits	8. Nuts	13. Shellfish
4. Legumes	9. Eggs	14. Meats
5. Fish, salt water	10. Dairy products	15. Processed meats

For vegetarians, the ranking is as follows (with the exception of eggs and dairy products, this also applies to vegans):

FOOD GROUP PRIORITIES: VEGETARIAN			
1. Vegetables	3. Legumes	5. Eggs	7. Nuts
2. Whole grains	4. Fruits	6. Dairy products	8. Seeds

✤ *Balance—Flavors and Colors*

The concept of the five flavors of food representing a balanced diet comes from the Laws of the Five Elements in traditional Oriental practice. According to this philosophy, each of the five flavors is associated with a different element and supports different organs and functions of our body.

In the Chinese philosophy, eating a variety of foods that contain these different flavors is an important part of a balanced diet. An excess or deficiency of a certain flavor can cause an imbalance of energy in the body and thus lead to specific symptoms and diseases. Excesses of salt and of sweet are two common examples; low intakes of bitter or sour foods may lead to other difficulties.

All the flavors are not necessarily eaten in equal proportions. The flavor focus may vary from season to season, as the elemental dominance changes, and according to our individual balance. There are many naturally sweet foods available, and these are consumed more plentifully than sour, salty, bitter, or spicy foods. Making a meal that contains all the five flavors is a challenge for any artful chef. The following table provides examples of foods associated with the different flavors.

Another way of viewing this balance is in terms of the colors of the foods, with a different element associated with each color. These colors may act like the flavors in stimulating certain organs and functions. Thus, the red foods, such as meats, cayenne pepper, and tomatoes, may stimulate blood and circulation; green foods, such as many vegetables, may help purify us and support metabolism or strengthen the liver. This view actually seems to have a physiological basis in many instances.

ELEMENTAL NUTRITION

Element	Wood	Fire	Earth	Metal	Water
Organs	Liver Gall Bladder	Heart Small Intestine	Spleen Stomach	Lungs Large Intestine	Kidneys Bladder
Color	Green	Red	Yellow	White	Blue/Black

Functions	Purification
	Metabolism
		Circulation
		Vitalization
			Digestion
			Distribution
				Elimination
				Mental
				  Circulation
					Storage
					Emotional
					  Circulation

Flavor	Sour	Bitter	Sweet	Spicy/Pungent	Salty
Foods	Lemons Other citrus Sauerkraut Pickles Vinegars Buttermilk Yogurt Preserved foods	Lettuce Spinach Chard Other greens Celery Asparagus Eggplant Some nuts Herbs	Grains Potatoes Carrots Beets Squash Peas Corn Yams Sweet potatoes Most fruits Sugar cane Honey Maple syrup Milk	Onions Garlic Radish Mustard Cayenne Chili pepper Horseradish Chives	Seaweed Ocean fish Celery Olives Salted foods Miso Capers Soy sauce Brine foods

❧ Balance—Acid-Alkaline

This concept, which I discuss more thoroughly in my first book, *Staying Healthy with the Seasons,* fits in well with many of the other aspects of a healthy diet. To put it simply, foods are classified as mainly acid or alkaline, not according to their taste but to the residue left after they have been metabolized in the body.

Our blood has a normal pH of 7.41 that is fairly stable. A diet that is too acidic affects our blood and tissues and creates congestion of mucus in different body areas.

Usually I suggest 70–80 percent alkaline and balanced foods in spring and summer months. During later autumn and winter, at least 65–70 percent alkaline and balanced foods would be all right. In very cold climates, a higher percentage of richer acid-forming foods may be tolerated, as these foods are higher in fats and burn hotter as body fuel. Also, fewer vegetables and far fewer fruits are available in winter and cold climates. By and large, whenever possible, we need lots of vegetables and whole grains to keep the body balanced.

ACID-ALKALINE FOODS

Alkaline	Balanced	Acid	
all vegetables	brown rice	wheat	butter*
most fruits	corn	oats	milk*
millet	soybeans	white rice	cheeses*
buckwheat	lima beans	pomegranates	eggs
sprouted beans	almonds	strawberries	meats
sprouted seeds	sunflower seeds	cranberries	fish
olive oil	Brazil nuts	breads	poultry
soaked almonds	honey	refined flour	
	most dried beans & peas	refined sugar	
	tofu	cashews, pecans,	
	vegetable oils	& peanuts	

*Some authors place milk products in the balanced area; I don't.

A REVIEW OF RECOMMENDED
DIETARY CHANGES

We know that we have our work cut out for us when we consider that it is very likely that the poor farming people of the "backward" nations have a better diet than we do. The American diet is far from the local seasonal vegetable-grain diet of less wealthy cultures. Instead of traditional fare, many of us dine regularly on prefabricated, processed, or treated foods with increased amounts of meat, fat, sugar, salt, and the many additives that help to flavor the refined foods.

With this all too popular American diet, there has been a huge decrease in the complex-carbohydrate fiber foods and in the natural high-vitamin/mineral whole foods, as well as deficiencies of the essential fatty acids, while intake of many unneessary and damaging fats have increased. The high amounts of refined oils (hydrogenated) and saturated fats can cause much disease. The decrease in the nutrition per calorie ratio with the increase in simple sugar and refined food intake has led to a strange combination of obesity and malnutrition. Many of our vital nutrients, such as vitamins A, C, and E, the B vitamins, calcium, magnesium, chromium, and zinc, may be missing from our diet. This is of special concern in teenagers and the elderly who tend to limit their diet more than other segments of the population.

A primary focus of this book is to help the reader shift his or her diet from the Standard American Diet (SAD) to a healthier one. For this we first need to reject the processed foods, high-fat foods, lunch meats, and high-sugar foods that are so prevalent. For example, many Americans are consuming close to half of their dietary calories as fats—nearly twice the level that is healthy. Nutritionist Jane Brody points out that additives, as well, are a dominant part of our consumption. The average American in recent years annually consumed 128 pounds of sugar, 15 pounds of salt, 9 pounds of 33 common additives, and 1 pound of the other 2,600 food additives, for a total of 153 pounds—yes, the average human weight—consumed yearly in mostly unnecessary, harmful ingredients.

Changing our diets may be a difficult task. It takes guts and a lot of work. Our cravings for fats, sweets, and processed foods are deeply ingrained. And our images are at stake: the meat-and-potatoes, beer-and-pretzel man could not possibly eat those sissy salads and health-nut foods such as rice and vegetables! Some of us still think we need our hunk of protein, but evidence to the contrary is building. Any of us who are reading or listening know that we have to get more basic and natural foods, and less salty and sweet or fatty foods, into our diet.

We need to begin by selecting healthful foods when shopping, when cooking, and in restaurants. We should not shop when hungry. When we do shop, we should skip many of the aisles with those fancy, colorful boxes and cans. This will help to eliminate many unnecessary and unwholesome foods. We want to choose foods as close to their natural state as possible.

Many authors suggest that these changes may decrease the death rates from cardiovascular disease and diabetes by 25–30 percent, and may also reduce the cancer rate. A diet such as this will most assuredly affect the vitality of newborn babies, the quality of our later years, and our longevity. The nationwide increase in chronic disease is primarily related to diet, and with more future-sighted vision, we can simultaneously grow both older and healthier.

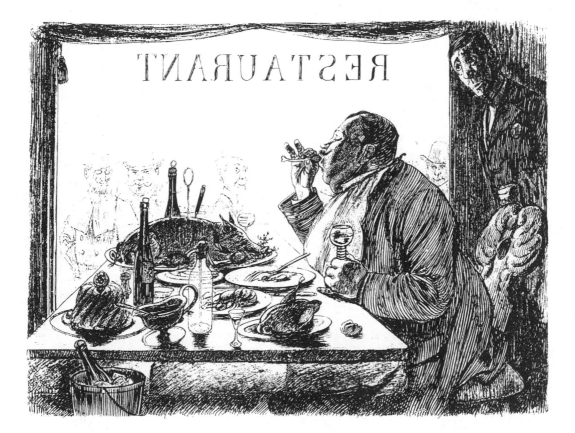

"Your Ideal Diet brings the freshest available foods from nature combined and prepared to meet the needs of your particular body, activity level, and state of health."

ELSON M. HAAS

CHAPTER 2

YOUR IDEAL DIET

Dare I even attempt to discuss "the Ideal Diet"? To call any one diet "the diet" is to misunderstand the basic aspects of nutrition and to mislead ourselves into believing that we can find one diet, stick with it forever, and not ever worry again about food. Instead, I will lay out several patterns, and discuss the basic foods that we can apply to these patterns.

The Ideal Diet is the individual diet that adapts and fluctuates with our needs. It will change with our activity levels, the state of our health, where we live, the time of the year, and even the daily weather. Let us assume that we are healthy and we expect this diet to maintain our good health. Learning to listen to our individual needs is vital to both maintaining and adapting our own correct diets. The biggest problem with this, of course, is that our current lifestyles and busy environments take us out of this sensitive mode, and most of us get caught up in what the technological society has to offer instead of creating what we need to nourish ourselves and our families. The essential food is already available, but it takes time to gather (shop) and prepare it, and we may not choose to take this time when we could be working or doing other things to support ourselves. We must realize that to create an Ideal Diet, we need to make nourishing ourselves a high priority, because without that basic support (good nutrition) for health and vitality, the rest of our life has less meaning. If we can momentarily step back from day-to-day existence and take an honest look at our lives, we will realize that simply dragging ourselves around to a job and working by caffeine stimulation lacks quite a bit. Learning to nourish the body to give it the best possible chance for optimum energy makes sense from the standpoint of physical productivity, mental clarity, and emotional contentment, and of religious-spiritual well-being, as the body is a holy temple to house the spirit.

Ideally, we want to obtain and consume (and even grow) the most wholesome, fresh, and organic (chemical-free) foods. Our meals should be simple in the number of foods we include, the amount we consume, and the way we combine them. Our diet also needs to vary in quantity and type of foods with our activity level, the local climate, and the time of year. And, of course, it should consist of the best foods available. Finding the freshest seasonal foods at our stores or local farmers' markets and creating our meals around them is a much better plan than the opposite approach of planning a meal and then searching for the appropriate foods.

As I have emphasized, in the long run, a diet centered around whole grains and vegetables will best serve us individually as well as contribute to greater planetary harmony. The whole grain-legume mixture with abundant vegetables, both cooked and raw, is the main diet of the majority of the Earth's people and, I think, the necessary beginning of our Ideal Diet. We must assume that following our instincts to nourish ourselves with what is available on our planet makes for the best diet. There is some order, I believe, to this universe, and we will have a lot less difficulty if we attune ourselves to that, as well as to our individual participation in it.

A GENERAL GUIDELINE FOR THE PROPORTIONS OF FOODS IN DIFFERENT TYPES OF DIETS

	Omnivore	*Lacto-Ovo-Vegetarian*	*Vegan*
Whole grains	25–30%	25–35%	30–40%
Vegetables	25–35	25–35	30–40
Legumes	5–10	10–15	10–15
Fruit	10–15	10–15	10–20
Nuts and seeds	5–10	5–10	10–15
Dairy products, eggs	5–10	10–15	
Meats, poultry, fish	10–15		

Here are some guidelines for the Ideal Diet:

1. **Produce**—5 or more servings per day of vegetables and fruits. Fresh is best.

2. **Starches**—4 or more servings per day of whole grains, potatoes, hard squashes.

3. **Proteins**—2–3 servings per day of sprouted legumes or seeds, cooked legumes, fish, eggs, seeds, nuts, poultry, lamb, beef, or pork—pretty much in that order of preference, in my opinion.

4. **Calcium foods**—2 or more servings per day, but no more than two of the dairy foods (if tolerated); fewer dairy foods is probably best. Calcium foods include nuts, seeds, and green leafy vegetables for any diet; milk, cheese, and yogurt for lacto-ovo or omnivore diets.

5. **Oils**—1 or 2 servings per day of vegetable oils. Olive, grape seed, flaxseed, canola, and sunflower oils are the best choices. Nuts and seeds will also provide some vitamin E and the essential fatty acids.

INDIVIDUAL NEEDS

How can we discern our individual dietary needs? First and foremost, we should listen to our bodies. If we have forgotten how to do this, we can relearn. But many people cannot or will not take the time or change their lives in order to reconnect with this instinctual process, so we need some basic guidelines. If we get the key concepts under our belt, the fine-tuning of our diet then really becomes the art and adventure of nutrition.

Besides listening to ourselves, it will do us well to listen to Nature. She is a great teacher and will provide us with the information and nourishment as we need it. Watching the seasons and the growing cycles of plants is the beginning. Working in a garden or planting our own food with family or friends is the best way to stay connected to the Earth and her secrets of health. When we do not eat from our gardens, we should be aware of where and how foods are produced, as well as how our bodies use and recycle them by digestion, assimilation, and elimination. Another way to support our individual needs is to be aware of our own states of health. The Ideal Diet discussed here is for those of us in basically good health who wish to maintain that state. It is usually a marked improvement over what we have been eating. It may reduce the incidence of many degenerative disease processes and support health by providing the required nutrients and normalize body weight over time, correcting the common obesity that results from the Standard American Diet. Furthermore, our digestive functions will improve, which is so important to overall health. Allergies to foods and the environment will likely diminish as we move away from refined foods and the overuse of wheat and cow's milk products.

Metabolic typing is based on the work of William Donald Kelley, a dentist who has made fairly deep investigations into nutrition. According to Dr. Kelley, there are three types of people or, more accurately, states of being, based on previous diet, activity, and life experience atop our basic nature. Each of us fits into one of these types according to whether we are dominated by one or the other of the two branches of our nervous system—the sympathetic and the parasympathetic—or whether we are in balance between them. Certain types of body chemistry are also associated with these states.

Most people are balanced types and need to create a balance between alkaline and acid foods. If we are healthy, our diets are usually more alkaline in spring and summer and slightly more acid in autumn and winter. Overall, the balanced healthy person needs to eat broadly from the wide range of natural foods. I believe, however, that we need to consume more alkaline-forming foods, at least 60 percent of the diet, all year round.

A sympathetic type is likely to have a more acid biochemistry, prone not only to subtle congestive problems, such as tension, constipation, or insomnia, but also to long-term degenerative diseases, such as atherosclerosis or hypertension. People with this biochemistry or temporary overbalance would do better on a more vegetarian or alkaline diet, which is also lower in protein and fat foods. Lots of fruits and vegetables can be consumed. Lighter eating is helpful for this metabolic type.

METABOLIC TYPES

Sympathetic *(Acid Body Chemistry)*	*Parasympathetic* *(Alkaline Body Chemistry)*
Action-oriented	Inaction-oriented
More nerve energy into energy production	More nerve energy into digestion and internal function
Intellectual	Intuitive
Fast or catabolic metabolism	Slower, anabolic metabolism
Lose weight easily, gain with difficulty	Gain weight easily, lose with difficulty
Prone to tension, constipation or insomnia	Prone to lethargy or diarrhea
Exercise-oriented	Exercise-avoidant
Energy improves with vitamin C	Little effect on energy with vitamin C
Minimal niacin reaction*	Big niacin reaction
Do better on alkaline diet	Need more acid diet

*The niacin reaction mainly involves heat flushing and tingling of the skin.

Alkaline, or parasympathetic-dominant, people need just the opposite type of diet to bring them back into balance. For these individuals, fasting can be disastrous, causing a worsening of fatigue and other symptoms. Eating a more acid diet, even meats and fish, will often help. A diet with higher levels of protein (and usually a little more fat) and more food overall, will help raise the energy level, and with it, the metabolism to handle this food.

Which type we are determines the relative amounts of acid and alkaline foods we need in our diet. The chart below lists foods according to these types.

ACID–ALKALINE FOODS

Alkaline		Neutral	Acid	
Fruits	Salt	Vegetable oils	Meat	Nuts
Vegetables	Herbs	Milk	Fish	Food additives
Sea vegetables	Spices	Cream	Eggs	Drugs
Millet	Wine	Butter	Beans	Liquor
Seeds		Cheese	Grains	
		Honey	(except millet)	

According to Dr. Kelley, we can adapt our basic diet of whole grains (slightly more acid) and vegetables (more alkaline) by using the other foods to shift to either a more acid or alkaline diet. With this knowledge, and if we are balanced, the time of year and our climate will suggest the predominant focus of our food choices.

If we are an acid type, and our diet tends toward more alkaline foods, we may still eat our richest foods in the winter. In the summer, however, we may fast occasionally or consume a much higher percentage of fruits, vegetables, and juices. If we are a more alkaline type, we need a more acid diet to fuel our body. Shifting with the seasons may allow us more fruits and vegetables in the spring and summer, while in the winter we need to get that warmth from the richer fuel of the meats, dairy products, beans, and nuts.

If we follow this plan, our health will improve, and we will move toward a balanced chemistry. Then we will need to shift our diets again to meet our new needs and to support our new energy states. Being healthy then becomes a process of continued awareness and adaptation to our ever-changing states of being. And that's when the fun begins!

CHANGING YOUR DIET

Eating seasonally provides you with foods from nature close to the time they are harvested and made available, and this gives you the most nourishment and vitality. Ideally, the natural flavors of the wholesome foods will be what appeals to and satisfies your palates and bodies. From day to day and season to season, the diet described here will also provide you with a variety of nutrients. It contains a balance of the food groups just discussed—protein foods, calcium foods, essential oils, produce, and starches—with the latter two the dominant groups. In this new diet, meals and snacks are simple, not combining a wide range of foods. There is a balance through the day, rather than at each meal. Eating fruits and sweet foods alone, as well as minimizing the combinations of starches and protein, will aid digestion and allow the best utilization of the nutrients from a wide variety of foods.

I suggest that you organize your daily diet according to the food groups that you will consume at certain times, while taking into account your day's activities, including exercise, work, and relaxation. A sample day's plan is presented below. Those with special work or sleep schedules or with varying types of productivity or cycles will have to adapt this plan to meet their schedules.

YOUR IDEAL DIET

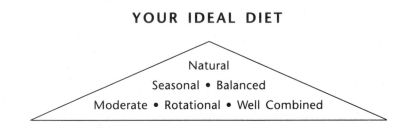

Natural
Seasonal • Balanced
Moderate • Rotational • Well Combined

Obviously, this diet will vary with the seasons and climate as well as your activity level and individual needs and metabolism. If you are trying to gain or lose weight, you will have to make modifications. If you are weight training, for example, and trying to increase your bulk and muscle mass, you will need bigger meals and more protein for dinner. If you want to drop some weight, eating a light dinner is probably the key (without later snacks), as well as eating moderately at all meals and increasing your physical activity. No kidding! It works if you actually do it.

Depending on your work schedules and specific metabolisms, you may want to switch the lunch and dinner meals (see menus in next chapter) and have your main meals at dinner instead of lunch. This will be discussed later in regard to the specific menu plans and recipes. Overall, it is healthier to consume more of your food earlier in the day when it can be digested and assimilated more completely, and to eat very lightly (if at all) after nightfall.

Now, I will go through a more complete example of a day's schedule for liquid and food intake, general activities, and other healthful tips.

SAMPLE DIET

Time of Day	Food	Examples	Portion	Reason
A.M. 6:00– 7:30 A.M.	Fruit	Orange or grapes	$^{1}/_{2}$–1 orange 10–20 grapes	A simple carbohydrate breaks our fast and kick-starts our engine/digestive tract.
Breakfast 7:00– 8:30 A.M.	Starch	Whole grain cereal or hard squash	1–2 bowls	A complex carbohydrate breakfast is our time-release energy capsule.
Snack 10:00– 11:00 A.M.	Nuts or seeds	Almonds or sunflower seeds	One handful	This fat/oil primes our engine and stimulates HCl and pancreatic enzymes, such as *lipase*.
Lunch 11:30– 1:00 P.M.	Protein and green vegetable	Chicken with broccoli, or spinach salad w/tomato and garbanzo sprouts	Moderation to satisfaction	This combination offers more nutrient/fuel intake and chlorophyll to further support digestion.
Snack 3:00– 4:00 P.M.	Fruit, vegetable, or starch	Apples, carrot sticks, or rice cakes	1 portion	A simple food to provide some energy lift for late afternoon.
Dinner 5:30– 7:00 P.M.	Starch and vegetable	Brown rice w/mixed vegetables or pasta primavera	Moderation to satisfaction	This basic complex carbohydrate meal provides energy and nourishment, and is light enough to allow proper digestion before bed.
Optional Snack 7:30– 9:00 P.M.	Fruit, vegetable, or starch	Apple and dates, celery, or popcorn	1 portion	A light snack if needed, depending on other foods consumed and individual metabolism.

DAILY SCHEDULE

✤ Morning ✤

- Arise from sleep with the sun. Go to sleep early enough to awaken without an alarm. Try to arise at least one hour before you must leave home.
- Sit quietly or lie propped up in bed and meditate and/or plan your day. Let any concerns or frustrations settle and visualize clearly how you would like to see your day.
- Drink two glasses of purified or spring water. One may have a quarter or half of a fresh lemon squeezed into it to help with morning purification.
- Do some stretches and light exercise.
- Eat a piece or two of fruit.
- A more vigorous exercise period may be included in this time period as well, either before or after fruit, depending upon your needs.
- Shower or bathe, and get ready for the day.
- A whole grain or starch breakfast (single or double portion) can be consumed within 30–60 minutes after the fruit. Some tea can be taken at this time or even with the fruit earlier.
- If supplements are taken, this can be done now.
- In an hour or two (midmorning, or 10:00–11:00 A.M.), a handful of one type of nut or seed may be consumed.
- More water or tea can follow, up to about half an hour before lunch.

MORNING NOTE: You have started your body slowly and moved into a work pace. You have taken several cups of liquids (not caffeine), done some exercise, cleaned and nourished your body, first with simple fruits, then more complex carbohydrates, followed with fat/oil-containing protein food. This allows early light eating and allows your digestive tract time to "break fast."

✤ Afternoon ✤

- The midday meal can be a substantial one to nourish you for the afternoon and may consist of a protein food and vegetables, including at least one green vegetable.

- A brief period (15–20 minutes) of relaxation and recharging may follow lunch. A short walk outdoors would be helpful as well to air out the brain, especially for indoor workers.

- Supplements can be taken at this time.

- A midafternoon snack may consist of a fruit, vegetable, or starch, or even a protein food, depending upon your needs and food organization plan.

- Later afternoon might include another cup of tea or a glass or two of water, in preparation for exercise.

- After work, some exercise or relaxation can be done, also depending on needs and previous activities. Your main exercise may be at this time, as it is for many individuals.

❧ EVENING ❧

- Dinner may consist of a starch and vegetables or a protein and vegetables.

- It is best to follow a good meal with a relaxation period.

- Supplements can also be taken at this time.

- Then some type of mild activity may aid digestion and assimilation. A short walk is a good idea, alone or with the kids, the dog, or a friend.

- The evening brings relaxation through reading; viewing a square box with moving, talking figures; working; or romancing, depending on your wishes. The evening is a good time to nourish yourself in other ways besides eating food.

- A light evening snack of a fruit, vegetable, or starch may be consumed. This is optional. Fruit may be preferred as it is sweet (a common flavor choice after dinner) and simple to digest.

- Some relaxing tea, warm lemon water, or a glass of plain water can be imbibed in the evening.

- Certain before-bed supplements, such as calcium/magnesium, can also be taken.

- A good night's sleep is now in order.

- Be aware of your dreams and open to remembering them in the morning to learn a little more about yourself.

DAILY DIETARY SCHEDULE

DIET ACTIVITY	POSSIBLE TIME	FOOD CHOICE
Preparation	6:00–7:00 A.M.	water
Breakfast	6:30–7:30 A.M.	fruit
Breakfast	7:30–8:30 A.M.	starch
Snack	10:00–11:00 A.M.	nut or seed
Lunch	12:00–1:00 P.M.	protein/vegetable
Snack	3:00–4:00 P.M.	fruit, vegetable, or starch
Dinner	5:30–7:00 P.M.	starch/vegetable or protein/vegetable
Snack	8:00–9:00 P.M.	fruit, vegetable, or starch

In food groups this is broken down into the following, depending, of course, on the size of portions consumed:

Breakfast	1–2 fruits, 1–2 starches
Morning snack	1 nut or seed (1 protein, 1 calcium, and 1 oil food)
Lunch*	1–2 proteins, 2–3 vegetables
Afternoon snack	1–2 vegetables or 1 fruit
Dinner*	1–2 starches or 1–2 proteins, and 2–3 vegetables
Evening Snack	1 fruit, 1 vegetable, or 1 starch

The breakdown of our "new" food groups gives us the following totals:

Produce	6–8 servings on the average
Starches	4–6 servings
Proteins	2–3 servings
Calcium foods	2–3 servings; includes green vegetables, nuts or seeds, and some protein foods
Oil foods	1–2 servings nuts/seeds and/or vegetable oil

---

*Fresh cold-pressed vegetable oil might also be consumed with lunch or dinner; in that case, add one oil food.

SUPPLEMENTS TO THE DIET

Even if we eat the Ideal Diet for an extended period of time, it is hard to maintain an entire balance of nutrients from day to day, and our utilization of the nutrients from these wholesome foods is dependent upon a generally healthy digestion and absorption and a minimum of stress or special, extra needs.

If we are healthy, with strong, consistent energy, and we sleep well, live in an unpolluted natural environment, do not hustle and bustle about to work and play, eat a variety of wholesome foods from the earth, and have good digestion and assimilation, we probably need very little, if any, supplements. If anything, extra minerals may be required, particularly those that might be deficient in the soils where we live.

However, most of us living in the latter twentieth century do not live or eat in this ideal fashion. We may eat on the run, drive on freeways, breathe in polluted air, drink contaminated water, come in contact with various chemicals, and have a lot on our minds. In other words, we have a lot of stimuli, stress, and energy needs.

Those of us who fit into this more realistic lifestyle category of today, I believe, need a stabilizing, nourishing program of vitamins, minerals, and other supplements. In this brief section, I suggest an optimum supplement plan to accompany a basically healthy diet for the average adult male or female with a mild amount of activity and stress. There are two columns in the accompanying chart: one for the suggested supportive intake level to supplement the basic diet, and the other to offer a possible daily intake range to take into account the various supplement preparations and individual variances.

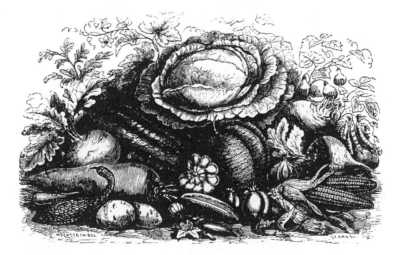

GENERAL ADULT INSURANCE DAILY SUPPLEMENT PROGRAM

Vitamin	Form	Suggested Daily Amount	Possible Range
Vitamin A	palmitate	5,000 IU	5,000–10,000 IU
Beta-Carotene	vegetable	15,000 IU	10,000–25,000 IU
Vitamin B_1	thiamine-HCl	15 mg	10–50 mg
Vitamin B_2	riboflavin	10 mg	10–50 mg
Vitamin B_3	niacin (preferred) or niacinamide	25 mg 50 mg	10–100 mg 10–100 mg
Vitamin B_5	calcium pantothenate	100 mg	50–100 mg
Vitamin B_6	pyridoxine-HCl or pyridoxal-5-phosphate	25 mg	10–100 mg
Vitamin B_{12}	cyanocobalamin or cobalamin	100 mcg	50–500 mcg
Folic acid	folacin	400 mcg	400–1,000 mcg
Biotin	biotin	250 mcg	150–500 mcg
PABA	para-aminobenzoic acid	50 mg	25–100 mg
Choline	choline bitartrate	500 mg	100–1,000 mg
Inositol	inositol	50 mg	10–200 mg
Bioflavonoids	mixed complex	250 mg	100–500 mg
Vitamin C	ascorbic acid	2,000 mg	500–3,000 mg
Vitamin D	D_3-ergocalciferol	400 IU	200–600 IU
Vitamin E	alpha tocopherol with mixed tocopherols	400 IU	200–600 IU
Vitamin K	phylloquinone	100 mcg	50–200 mcg

The amounts suggested are usually at or above the RDA but not at the much higher levels that might be suggested for a more stressed or imbalanced, symptomatic individual or that might be used in specific therapeutic situations. Remember, this insurance formula is for the basically healthy man or woman.

Mineral	Form	Suggested Daily Amount	Possible Range
Calcium	dicalcium phosphate or calcium aspartate or citrate	600 mg	500–1,200 mg
Magnesium	oxide, citrate, or aspartate	500 mg	300–750 mg
Potassium	chloride	400 mg	100–1,000 mg
Iron	citrate or chelate	15 mg	10–18 mg
Zinc	sulfate, gluconate, or picolinate	30 mg	15–45 mg
Copper	sulfate or chelate, such as gluconate	2 mg	1–3 mg
Iodine	potassium iodide	150 mcg	50–200 mcg
Manganese	sulfate or chelate	10 mg	2–10 mg
Selenium	selenomethionine or sodium selenite	200 mcg	50–200 mcg
Chromium	amino acid chelate, oxide, or picolinate	200 mcg	50–500 mcg
Silicon	equisetum-horsetail	20 mg	10–50 mg
Molybdenum	sodium molybdate or chelate	200 mcg	50–200 mcg
Vanadium	pentoxide or chelate	200 mcg	50–200 mcg

Other possibilities:

Flaxseed oil (OR)	Balanced omega-3 and omega-6 combination	2 tsp or 4 capsules	1–3 tsp 3–6 capsules
Omega-3 fatty acids	EPA and DHA oil capsules	1,000 mg	500–1,500 mg
Lactobacilli cultures	powder or capsules	1 billion count	50 million to 10 billion organisms per dose

NOTE: Supplements should be hypoallergenic—not made from milk, yeast, wheat, corn, or soy—and contain no sugar, preservatives, or artificial colors.

"Using recipes as inspiration instead of rigid structures will allow your creativity to express itself and make cooking and eating more joyful experiences."

ELEONORA MANZOLINI

CHAPTER 3

BASICS FOR THE IDEAL DIET

Before the recipes, menu plans, and seasonal food lists in the upcoming chapters, Eleonora and I have included some "kitchen basics:" cooking and storing ideas and some general tips and shortcuts. We hope all of this information will help you on your path to a new way of eating, or will allow you to fine-tune your already health-oriented diet. Enjoy!

❖ Kitchen Basics

Washing grains: I like the swirling method I learned from cookbook author Annemarie Colbin. It is more effective than running water over the grains in a colander. Put the grains in a bowl and cover with twice the amount of water. Swirl thoroughly and pour off all the floating debris and stray grains. Catch the rest in a colander. If the water is very dirty, repeat the procedure. Quinoa, amaranth, and millet need to be washed more carefully, several times at least.

Cooking grains: The following are some cooking times and grain-to-water ratios for the more commonly utilized grains.

Brown rice: Combine 1 cup rice to 2 cups cold water and a pinch of salt. The salt is important even if you are on a salt-free diet because it brings out the full flavor of the grain. Bring to a boil, adjust the flame to low, cover, and cook the rice for 50–60 minutes. If you are making rice with steamed vegetables, you can lay the cut up vegetables on top of the rice during the last 10 minutes and they will cook with the steam from the rice. Rice connoisseurs suggest cooking the rice undisturbed for 1 hour over a low heat. The pot must have a tight seal so the steam does not escape, and to tell it's done, listen to the pot; it will stop bubbling and you will hear a slight crackling or popping sound of rice toasting. Many rice lovers will also prepare the rice with more salt, about 1/4–1/2 teaspoon per cup of uncooked rice, and 1/2–1 tablespoon of oil or butter.

Barley: Cook with the same amount of water as you would rice. I have found it takes slightly longer, 60–70 minutes. Or you can soak it first for one hour, then cook for 15–20 minutes.

Quinoa: ("Keenwa") 1 cup of quinoa to 2 cups of water and a pinch of salt. Cover, bring to a boil, and simmer 15 minutes.

Millet: Another trick I learned from Annemarie Colbin is to dry-roast this grain in a cast-iron or stainless steel skillet until a few grains begin to pop, about 5–10 minutes. Then add 2 cups of water for each cup of millet and the usual pinch of salt. Cover, bring to a boil, lower the heat and simmer for about 30–40 minutes. Fluff with fork before serving. If just cooking millet in water, rinse it well to remove any unseen dirt.

Kasha: Bring 2 cups of water and a pinch of salt to a boil. Add 1 cup of kasha, lower the flame, and simmer for 15–20 minutes.

You may wish to use a pressure cooker for some grains in order to shorten the cooking time. Do not cook millet, quinoa, oats, or any cracked grain in the pressure cooker since it may clog up the escape valve and cause an explosion. Pressure-cooked grains have a totally different texture and taste, especially rice, which tends to stick together. It is wonderful for making sushi, but not appropriate for a rice salad or pilaf.

GRAIN/WATER PROPORTIONS AND COOKING TIMES

Brown rice	1:2	50–60 minutes
Millet	1:2	30–40 minutes
Oats, rolled	1:2	15–20 minutes
Kasha	1:2–2 1/2	15–20 minutes
Barley	1:2 1/2	1 hour
Couscous	1:2	soak 10 minutes in boiling water

Washing and soaking beans: Beans that are bought in bulk need picking over since they often contain stones. The worst are red lentils and I suggest that you do not buy them in bulk, but get the already cleaned and packaged ones.

The following beans do not need soaking: all kinds of lentils, split peas, and adzuki beans. All other beans are best soaked overnight in twice the amount of water. This will shorten their cooking time. Throw away the soaking water to reduce the gas-producing effects. If you do not have time to soak the beans overnight, you can use a quick method. Boil them in twice the amount of water for 5 minutes and then let them sit covered for 1 hour; then change water for further cooking.

Cooking beans: Black-eyed peas, lima beans, small white/navy beans and adzuki beans can be cooked together with rice in the same pot since they have similar cooking times. Just add more water.

Pressure-cooking reduces the time by about one half, but be careful not to cook lentils and split peas in a pressure cooker since they may clog the escape valve and cause the pressure cooker to explode.

BEANS/WATER PROPORTIONS AND COOKING TIMES*

Red lentils	1:2	15–20 minutes
Lentils and split peas	1:2–2$\frac{1}{2}$	$\frac{1}{2}$ hour
Black-eyed peas, lima beans, mung beans, navy beans, adzuki beans, black beans	1:3	1 hour
Kidney beans, pinto beans, soybeans	1:3$\frac{1}{2}$	1$\frac{1}{2}$ hours
Garbanzo beans	1:4	2 hours

* Times are for unsoaked beans; if soaked overnight, cooking time is reduced by one–third.

Always salt your beans at the end, about 10 minutes before they are done. This is important since adding salt at the beginning will cause the beans to remain tough. If you prefer not to use salt, remember that beans cooked with no salt at all tend to disintegrate. This may be okay for soups and stews, but not if you are making a bean salad.

Beans, like grains, can be slow-cooked in an oven or crockpot. Place beans and water (add additional cup of water per additional cup of beans) in ovenproof bean pot or casserole dish. Put covered dish in oven and cook overnight or all day at low setting, 200°F–220°F. The beans will be more tasty, tender, and thicker than if you use the quicker cooking method.

For more flavorful, spicy beans, cook with lightly sautéed onion and garlic. Dice a large onion and a few cloves of garlic and lightly sauté with 2 teaspoons of canola or other light oil in the cooking pot. Add 2 cups of beans and about 6 cups of water, and simmer until the beans are tender. Optionally, to avoid the oil sauté, just add all the ingredients to the pot and cook.

To enhance and vary the flavor of beans, a variety of herbs and spices can be added to the cooking pot at the start or midway. If beginning with 2 cups of beans, try one or more of the following at your inspiration and taste:

SEASONINGS FOR BEANS

Vegetables	*Dried Herbs*	*Fresh Herbs*
garlic, 2–4 cloves	bay leaf, 1 or 2	cilantro, 4–6 teaspoons
onion, 1 medium or large	oregano, $1/2$ teaspoon	parsley, 2–3 sprigs
carrot, 1 or 2 chopped	basil, $1/2$–1 teaspoon	sage, 2–3 leaves
bell pepper, 1 chopped	cumin, 1–2 teaspoons	rosemary, 1 sprig
jalapeño, 1 sliced, seeded	cayenne, $1/4$ teaspoon	thyme, 2 sprigs
tomatoes, 2 fresh chopped	chili powder, $1/2$–1 teaspoon	
	sage, pinch	
	rosemary, $1/4$ teaspoon	
	thyme, $1/4$–$1/2$ teaspoon	

Cleaning vegetables: If you buy your root vegetables, such as carrots, radishes, and turnips from organic sources, there is no need to peel them; just scrub them with a stiff brush. Vegetables from commercial sources most of the time have been waxed and treated with chemical pesticides and therefore need peeling.

To peel tomatoes, drop them in boiling water for 10–15 seconds. Allow to cool and the skin will come off very easily.

To peel garlic, place your knife flat on the garlic clove and whack with your other hand. The covering will burst open and the clove can be easily removed.

For leafy greens, cut off the root end and plunge into a sink full of cold water. Swirl around a few times and let sit for awhile. The sand, dirt, and other debris will settle to the bottom, and the leaves will float to the top and can be removed. Repeat the procedure if the greens (such as spinach) are very dirty.

Some tips about fish: When buying a whole fish, make sure it has firm flesh, red gills, and bright eyes. Steaks or fillets should be moist and not flaky. It is a good idea to get your fish from a dependable source, not a supermarket, since it is often dipped in a solution of nitrites and nitrates to cover up any smell. Many stores also lay the fish on paper that is saturated with chemicals to preserve the color. Before cooking, it is best to rinse the fish under cold running water. Do not use a wooden cutting board for chopping up fish or meat, since the wood absorbs the juices and becomes a breeding ground for bacteria.

Seasoning: By seasoning, I don't mean just salt, even if it is a very important ingredient. I like to use sea salt, which is free of additives, and use it only in cooking, not at the table.

Herbs and spices can lend a great deal of taste to even the simplest dish, but it is important to use just the right amount that will enhance and not overpower the food. This is especially true for strong flavors such as garlic, cayenne, sage, and tarragon. It is best to start with a little and add more if necessary. For best results, fresh herbs should be added at the end of the cooking time, while dried herbs should be added at the beginning. Cayenne and freshly ground black pepper can be added individually at the table, since not everybody likes a very hot taste.

Here are some suggestions if you end up with too much of anything.

- *too salty:* Wash off the salt, or add oil or butter. When cooking grains or pasta, if the water is too salty, add a whole potato.
- *too sweet:* Add salt or increase the liquid.
- *too bitter:* Avoid salt and add something sweet.
- *too spicy:* Add potato or grain, or something sweet.
- *too sour:* Add salt or liquid.

For giving basic dishes like rice, vegetables, or chicken an international flavor, a simple seasoning list might include the following:

- *Italian:* basil, oregano, thyme, marjoram, garlic, olive oil
- *Chinese:* ginger, soy sauce, cayenne or chili oil, scallions, toasted sesame oil
- *Mexican:* cumin, cilantro, cayenne and chili pepper, garlic, salsa
- *Indian:* curry, coriander, cumin, saffron, cardamom, ghee (clarified butter)
- *French:* dill, tarragon, thyme, rosemary, mustard, butter, wine
- *Eastern European:* paprika, poppy seed, caraway, dill, onion, sour cream

Seasoning Mix

A general seasoning mixture can be made from your own favorite choices or from the following recipe of dried ingredients:

1–2 teaspoons sea salt

1–2 teaspoons onion powder

1/2 teaspoon garlic powder

1/2–1 teaspoon mustard

1/4–1/2 teaspoon cayenne powder or 1 teaspoon paprika

1/2 teaspoon kelp (optional)

2 teaspoons basil flakes

1 teaspoon parsley flakes

1/2 teaspoon thyme

1/2 teaspoon marjoram

1/2 teaspoon celery seeds

1/2 teaspoon curry (optional)*

---

* If using curry, replace thyme and marjoram with cumin and cardamom.

❖ A Few Tips and Shortcuts

- Soak beans overnight to cut cooking time; throw away soaking water.

- Soak nuts and seeds overnight, and they will become crunchier and easier to digest because the fats in them become more available as fatty acids. Soaked nuts and seeds also make wonderful additions to salads and can be stored in the refrigerator for a few days.

- Pressure-cooking beans and grains cuts the cooking time by approximately one-third. I like to pressure-cook a big batch of beans, and then store it in the freezer in small containers, just about enough for two people. In this way I can prepare a bean dish in no time at all, and besides, freezing helps get rid of the aspects that cause flatulence in many people.

- Wash salad and other leafy greens when you buy them; pat them dry, and then keep them in plastic bags in the vegetable compartment of the refrigerator so you do not have to waste a lot of time when you want to use them. I also like to chop the basic vegetables, like onions, garlic, carrots, celery, and parsley, and keep them ready to use in sealed containers in the refrigerator.

- Keep a few basic sauces ready in the refrigerator, such as tomato sauce. Just simmer fresh or canned peeled tomatoes for about 20 minutes with a little salt. You can then sauté onion, garlic, celery, carrot, parsley, and a little chili pepper in a small amount of olive oil, and add it to the tomatoes. It takes about 5 minutes to put the whole thing together. Store in plastic or stainless steel, not in aluminum or pottery ware.

- Miso/tahini mixture is also a basic condiment that keeps well. Just blend miso and tahini with a little rice vinegar and water. You can add garlic, ginger, or mustard to it to make it different every time, and use it as a salad dressing by adding more water, and as a dip or creamy sauce over grains if you keep it thicker.

- Flavored oils add zest to any dish. Being Italian, I am partial to olive oil, but you can use any oil you like. Make small bottles and add a different herb to each, i.e. garlic, hot chili pepper, tarragon, sage, rosemary, thyme, etc.

- If you do not have time to marinate things, here is a way to quick marinate. Bring your marinade to a boil and drop whatever you want to marinate into it for a few minutes.

- Instant pizza can be made by using tortillas or pita bread. Place them in the oven for a few minutes to crisp, spoon on some tomato sauce, your favorite toppings, and a little grated cheese, and put them into the oven again until the cheese melts.

- Quick-cooking grains are couscous, kasha, quinoa, and polenta.

- Frozen grapes and cherries make wonderful alternatives to candy, or as "ice cubes" for drinks.

- Almost any juices, fresh or bottled, can be placed in popsicle containers and frozen to make warm-weather treats for children of all ages.

- For thickening sauces and gravies, there are many substitutes for wheat flour. Equivalents to one tablespoon of wheat flour include half-tablespoons of arrowroot powder, rice or potato flour, or cornstarch.

- For those avoiding salt, lower sodium substitutes include kelp, regular or low-sodium tamari, light miso, lemon juice, ume vinegar, celery salt, various vegetable "salts," and the Seasoning Mix on page 44.

❧ *For Those Who Wish to Avoid Fats*

- Substitute fish, chicken, or vegetable stock for half or for the whole amount of oil called for in a recipe.

- Water-sauté food instead of stir-frying it in oil. Put about ½ to 1 cup of water or stock into a wok or skillet and bring it to a rapid boil. Quickly add vegetables and keep stirring over a high flame until done.

- Onions sautéed in their own juice and puréed with light miso make a wonderful onion butter which is great on toast or bread in place of real butter. The same thing can be done with most vegetables. See pages 71 and 72 for examples.

- Apple butter is a great no-fat spread for those with a sweet tooth.

- Purée a very loose oatmeal (about 1 cup of rolled oats or brown rice to 4 cups of water). Use instead of milk to make cream soups, gravies, and any dish which calls for milk.

- Tofu puréed with lemon juice makes a great mock sour cream. Also see recipes on pages 66 and 67.

❧ *About Storing*

- Cooked grains may be kept in a porcelain or wooden bowl in a cool place but out of the refrigerator. Covered with a napkin, they will keep for about 3 days. In the refrigerator they should be stored in airtight containers or they will absorb the flavor of other foods.

- Beans can be kept in jars on shelves or inside a cupboard. Cooked beans are best stored in the freezer in small containers.

- Mushrooms should be kept in a brown paper bag in the vegetable compartment of the refrigerator.

- Fresh herbs keep best in a glass of water in the refrigerator.

- Oils once opened should be refrigerated. The only exception is olive oil which should be kept in a dark place.

- Nuts and seeds are best refrigerated or even frozen.

- Flour should be kept in the refrigerator or freezer.

- Fruits, potatoes, tomatoes, onions, and garlic are best not refrigerated, but kept in a basket in a shady place or in a pantry.

CHAPTER 4

RECIPES FOR ALL SEASONS

Here are some basic recipes that can be used in all seasons, or adapted to suit your particular taste. Since grains, beans, and vegetables are what we believe to be the building blocks of a healthy diet, we have chosen recipes along these lines that can be prepared ahead of time and used in a variety of different ways. For instance, a quick lunch on a warm day could consist of a couple of slices of fresh crusty bread with a drizzle of olive oil, topped with *Salsa,* and a salad with *Low-Fat, Low-Salt Vinaigrette.* The *Steamed Vegetable Platter* could be puréed and used as a sauce for pasta or rice. The *Rainbow Rice* and *Chop Suey* are meals by themselves, and by varying the vegetables according to the seasons, they can be different each time. And of course, it is always a good idea to have a homemade *Tomato Sauce* in the refrigerator for a quick pasta, pizza, chicken, or fish dish.

We have also included some recipes here for those with special needs and/or interests: Wheat-Free, Milk/Egg-Free, Butter-Free Spreads, Seed Cheese and Yogurt (Dairy-Free and Raw), and Special Snacks for Kids.

It is our philosophy that "simple is best," and with a little planning ahead, a few basic ideas, and your own imagination, it will be easy and fun to create healthy, balanced meals for yourself and your family.

SOME BASIC RECIPES

Dr. Sun's Granola

6 cups rolled oats

2 cups almonds, chopped

1 cup chopped walnuts or peanuts (optional)

2 cups sunflower seeds

1 cup safflower or soy oil

$^1/_2$–$^3/_4$ cup maple syrup or honey

1–1$^1/_2$ tablespoons vanilla

1 tablespoon cinnamon (fresh ground is best)

$^1/_2$ teaspoon almond extract (optional)

1 teaspoon sea salt

1 cup dried, chopped apricots
  (organic, unsulfured, sun-dried are best)

1 cup raisins, currants, or chopped dates

▼ *Makes 12 cups*

Preheat oven to 325°F.

Mix oats, nuts, and seeds into large bowl. Lightly heat other ingredients, except dried fruit, in a saucepan, and then pour over oat mixture, tossing thoroughly. Spread this mix onto cookie sheet or baking pan. Bake for about 20 minutes, stirring granola occasionally, until evenly toasted. Let cool and then toss in large bowl with dried fruit (if you like the chewy component in your granola). Store properly in closed containers. Use as a snack or a cereal.

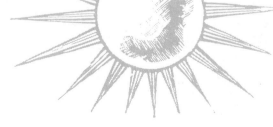

General Salad Ingredients

mixed lettuce (red or green leaf, butter,
   or romaine)

head lettuce, shredded

spinach, broken

green or red bell pepper, diced

carrots, sliced or grated

cabbage, red or green, shredded

mushrooms, wiped and sliced

green onions, sliced

alfalfa sprouts

bean sprouts (mung, green peas, garbanzo,
   or adzuki)

sunflower seeds

▼ *Limit to 4–6 choices*

Any green should be washed carefully and dried. Remove spinach stems. The sprouts, sunflower seeds, and mushrooms add some protein to the vegetable salad. Toss with a salad dressing of your choice.

Mixed Sprout Salad

1 cup each very fresh alfalfa, lentil, and
   mung bean sprouts

$^1/_2$ cup adzuki, green pea, or garbanzo sprouts or
   a mixed bean preparation

2 tablespoons sunflower seeds

$^1/_2$ cup chopped green onions

$^1/_2$ cup diced green pepper or cucumber

1–2 tablespoons chopped fresh herbs (optional), or
   1 tablespoon dried salad herbs

2 ripe tomatoes or 12 cherry tomatoes

▼ *Serves 4–6*

Toss ingredients together and then decorate with tomatoes. Serve with a dressing of olive oil, lemon juice, and salad herbs, or a dressing of your choice. This high-protein, nutritious salad is very filling.

Cold Rice Salad Variation

6 cups cooked brown rice

1 cup green and/or red pepper

4 green onions, chopped

4 radishes, sliced

$1/2$ cup fresh parsley, chopped

$1/2$ cucumber, peeled and diced (optional)

$1/2$ cup roasted sunflower seeds

8–10 lettuce leaves

2 cups alfalfa sprouts

2 tomatoes, sliced

1 whole lemon, wedged

▼ *Serves 6*

Mix rice with pepper, onions, radish, parsley, cucumber, and sunflower seeds. Place rice mixture in center of lettuce leaves, surround with alfalfa sprouts, and top with sliced tomatoes. If desired, sprinkle with salad herbs. Serve with lemon wedges. An olive oil vinaigrette or a nonfat yogurt vinaigrette make ideal dressings.

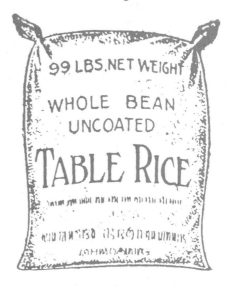

Low-Fat, Low-Salt Vinaigrette

This variation of a recipe from Dr. Dean Ornish's Stress, Diet, and Your Heart *is a healthy and tasty vinaigrette. There are even some decent oil-free dressings available in most stores.*

2 tablespoons oil (safflower, sunflower, or olive oil)

1–2 ounces vinegar (rice or apple cider) or
$^1/_2$–1 lemon, juiced

1–2 cloves garlic, minced or pressed

$^1/_2$ teaspoon dried mustard

$^1/_4$ teaspoon dried tarragon, $^1/_2$ teaspoon salad herbs,
or 1 teaspoon chopped fresh herbs

$^1/_4$ teaspoon dried basil or marjoram

$^1/_2$ cup nonfat yogurt, unsalted tomato juice, or water

pepper to taste

▼ *Makes about 1 cup*

Mix the ingredients together well, or place in blender for a short blend (15–30 seconds) on low speed. Achieve desired thickness with water.

Joe Terry's Miso Magic Dressing

This is also a low-fat and cholesterol-free, yet spicy and flavorful dressing for salads or other dishes, such as grains or vegetables. It needs a long, slow blender ride to make it really creamy and mix all the flavors.

3–4 cloves garlic

$^1/_4$ cup balsamic vinegar

$^1/_2$ cup water

$^1/_4$ cup white miso, unpasteurized

1 teaspoon prepared mustard

$^1/_8$ cup olive oil (optional)

▼ *Makes about 1$^1/_2$ cups*

Blend garlic cloves in vinegar and water. Slowly add miso, mustard, and olive oil.

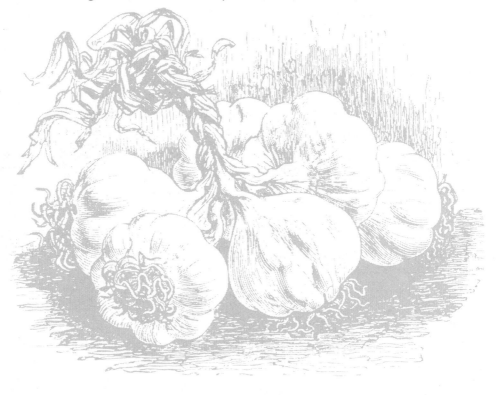

Vegetable Broth

2 cups potatoes, cut in small chunks

1–2 zucchinis, sliced

2 cups green cabbage, sliced (and/or other greens,
    such as spinach or kale)

1 large onion, sliced top to bottom

2 carrots, medium, sliced

1 clove garlic, minced

$1/2$ teaspoon sea salt

2 teaspoons olive oil

cayenne or black pepper, pinch or to taste

10–12 cups purified water

3–6 shiitake mushroom stems (optional)

▼ *Serves 6–8*

Slowly simmer all ingredients in a covered pot for an hour or more. Shiitake mushrooms will give a richer flavor to the broth; remove stems from soup when done.

For vegetable soup, cook the harder vegetables first, then add zucchini, cabbage and/or greens. For a thicker soup, add a cup of yellow or green split peas (see also *Thick (Spicy) Vegetable Soup*, p. 55). Other herbs and spices can be used if you wish. Blend part or all of cooled soup for a thicker broth or a rich soup. Serve soup with chopped green onion or cilantro, or eat vegetables and save broth for other recipes, such as for sauces or gravies.

NOTE: Eleonora likes to keep the scraps from onions, carrots, celery, and other vegetables in a plastic bag in the freezer until she has enough to make a vegetable stock. Then she simmers all of it with a strip of kombu seaweed and uses this broth as a base for other soups or for cooking grains.

Thick (Spicy) Vegetable Soup

1 pound small or medium potatoes,
  or cauliflower pieces

4 cups water

$^1/_4$ teaspoon cayenne, or to taste (optional for spicy)

$^1/_2$ teaspoon dried basil

$^1/_2$ teaspoon cumin

3 tablespoons sesame oil or corn oil
  (for a buttery flavor)

$^1/_2$–1 teaspoon sea salt

1 small onion, chopped

2 cloves garlic, chopped (optional)

$^1/_2$ cup tomato, diced

$^1/_2$ cup each of several of the following vegetables:
  carrot, celery, green pepper, zucchini, broccoli,
  cauliflower, beets (for pink soup)

$^1/_2$ cup green onions, chopped

▼ *Makes 5–6 cups*

Scrub and wash potatoes or cauliflower and boil in 4 cups water in a medium-sized pot or saucepan for 15–20 minutes. Allow to cool a bit, and blend with the water in which they were cooked, adding the seasonings, the oil, and the salt. Rinse vegetables, and chop into bite-sized pieces. Place the blended mixture and chopped vegetables into the pot or saucepan, cover, and cook over a low heat for 10–15 minutes. Top with green onions and serve.

For a specific vegetable soup, such as potato or broccoli, use primarily that vegetable. For a cream soup, use milk (preferably low-fat), or for a milk-free cream soup, blend in an appropriate amount (1 cup in this recipe) of well-cooked, moist oatmeal.

Salsa

3 cups chopped tomatoes, ripe

$^1/_2$ small onion, chopped

1 small jalapeño or chili pepper,
   seeds removed ($^1/_4$ cup chopped
   bell pepper for milder salsa)

2 cloves garlic, minced

$^1/_2$ teaspoon chili powder or
   $^1/_4$ teaspoon cayenne

2 teaspoons fresh lemon or
   lime juice

2 tablespoons chopped cilantro
   (optional)

$^1/_4$–$^1/_2$ teaspoon cumin
   (optional)

$^1/_4$ teaspoon salt (optional)

$^1/_2$ teaspoon oregano (optional)

▼ *Makes 3–4 cups*

Chop everything and mix. For a creamier salsa, purée in blender or food processor.

Guacamole

3 medium avocados

1 small tomato, chopped and
   drained (optional)

2 green onions, chopped fine
   (optional)

$^1/_4$ cup of Spanish, Bermuda, or
   yellow onion, diced (optional)

2 cloves garlic, minced

$^1/_2$ lemon or 1 lime, juiced

$^1/_4$ teaspoon cayenne or
   chili powder, or to taste,
   or small jalapeño pepper,
   finely chopped, seeds
   removed

$^1/_4$ –$^1/_2$ teaspoon salt, or to taste

▼ *Serves 4*

Mash avocados in a bowl, and mix in other ingredients. Serve cold with chips and salsa or with vegetables. Add water and lemon to make avocado salad dressing in blender. Add miso paste to taste for miso-avocado dressing. Blend in a block of tofu (with more water) for avocado-tofu dip or dressing. A simple guacamole will use only avocados, lemon, and salt. For a creamy version, add yogurt or sour cream.

Tostadas

(tortilla meals)

tortillas, corn or wheat

grains

refried beans

cheese, grated (jack, cheddar, cottage, or soy)

chopped onion

sprouts or iceberg lettuce, shredded

avocado slices or guacamole (p. 56)

black olives

salsa (p. 56)

sour cream (optional)

Oil skillet and heat (on low) one side of tortilla. Turn and spoon in grain or refried beans, sprinkle with cheese, and cover skillet to melt. Serve with toppings. For a taco, fold in half and heat, flipping to other half if necessary. Remove and add vegetable ingredients and seasonings of choice.

Steamed Veggie Platter

Use several or all of the following vegetables:

new potatoes, unpeeled

carrots, half-length strips

beets, quartered

broccoli florets with a little stem

cauliflower florets

zucchini, steamed whole, then sliced lengthwise

Steam vegetables until only slightly soft, about 10–15 minutes (zucchini, 5 minutes). Arrange all on a platter and season with melted butter or olive oil, lemon juice, and salt or herb seasoning. Garnish with cherry tomatoes if available. May also serve around a bowl with an herbal butter or any dip of your choice. Raw celery sticks, carrot sticks, and tomatoes can be used as well. In summer, a lightly steamed vegetable platter really brings out the natural flavors.

Sesame Salt (Gomasio)

sesame seeds

sea salt

A tasty seasoning for soup, salads, or grain and vegetable dishes. Roast sesame seeds in a dry skillet, stirring continuously, until a few begin to pop. Blend with sea salt, 1 part salt to 8–10 parts sesame seeds. Place in closed container and use as table seasoning.

Rainbow Rice

$^1/_2$ cup onion, chopped

$^1/_2$ cup red pepper, chopped

$^1/_2$ cup carrot, chopped

$^1/_2$ cup yellow squash, chopped

$^1/_2$ cup zucchini, chopped

$^1/_2$ cup purple (red) cabbage, chopped
  (or beet or eggplant)

$^1/_4$ cup green onions, chopped

2 tablespoons sunflower oil
  (or sesame, olive, or canola)

2 teaspoons soy sauce, or to taste

$^1/_2$ cup water

6 cups cooked rice

1 cup parsley, chopped, without stems

cayenne to taste (optional)

▼ *Serves 6–8*

Cut vegetables lengthwise and then dice. Sauté the vegetables in oil in this order: onion, pepper, squashes, cabbage (or eggplant or beet), and green onions, stirring and adding water and soy sauce. Add cooked rice in clumps, stir into vegetables, and heat gently for 5 minutes. Leave covered and serve warm. Before serving, add parsley (and cayenne if desired). This salad is good cold, and even better with a tofu or miso-tahini dressing (see seasonal recipes).

Chop Suey

$^1\!/_2$ cup oil (soy, canola, or sesame,
toasted optional)

1 cup green pepper, diced (or celery, sliced)

1 cup onion, sliced in crescents

2 cups button mushrooms, sliced top to bottom

1 cup water chestnuts, sliced

2 cups green cabbage, shredded

1 cup Napa or Chinese cabbage, shredded

1 cup bok choy

2 cups mung bean sprouts

3 cups water

$^1\!/_2$ cup arrowroot powder

$^1\!/_2$ cup soy sauce

cayenne pepper or chili oil to taste (optional)

6–8 cups cooked rice

1 cup raw or toasted almonds, slivered or chopped
(optional)

▼ *Serves 8–10*

Use a heavy, large skillet or a wok for this chop suey dish. Heat wok or skillet first on medium heat. Add oil and then immediately add the vegetables, at 1–2 minute intervals, first adding pepper and onions, then the mushrooms and water chestnuts, then greens, and then bean sprouts, adding splashes of water up to 1 cup as needed. Have ready, mixed together in a bowl, the arrowroot (a thickener), soy sauce, cayenne or chili oil if desired, and 1–2 cups cool water (until powder is dissolved). Stir liquid into vegetables, cover, and remove from heat. Serve over rice; it's nice.

If toasted almonds are desired, bake in oven on cookie sheet for 15–20 minutes at 300°F, or buy roasted almonds at the store. For additional flavor, sprinkle some tamari soy sauce over almonds before roasting.

Additional foods to add or substitute in this Chinese meal are: tofu in cubes, bamboo shoots, snowpeas, green beans, celery, green onions, sliced carrots, broccoli florets, cauliflower, zucchini, and minced garlic or ginger, or just any "interesting" veggies on hand. Also, a sukiyaki dish can be made in a pot using about half the portions of above ingredients and about a cup or more water, leaving out the almonds, substituting carrots for the green pepper, and adding some clear rice noodles and chunks of tofu. Simmer about 10 minutes, then add the greens, mung sprouts, and the arrowroot powder. For a little richer flavor, sauté the hard vegetables lightly in oil before adding to pot.

§ § § §

Here are three basic recipes for some common tomato sauces from a very useful recipe book, *The New Laurel's Kitchen*, by Laurel Robertson, Carol Flinders, and Brian Ruppenthal, published by Ten Speed Press.

Homemade Ketchup

We like this ketchup better than store-bought. It's free of additives and sugar, much lower in salt—and cheap.

1 12-ounce can tomato paste

$^1/_2$ cup cider vinegar

$^1/_2$ cup water

$^1/_2$ teaspoon salt

1 teaspoon oregano

$^1/_8$ teaspoon cumin

$^1/_8$ teaspoon nutmeg

$^1/_8$ teaspoon pepper

$^1/_2$ teaspoon mustard powder

squeeze of garlic from press

▼ *Makes 1$^3/_4$ cups*

Mix all ingredients together. Store in a jar in the refrigerator.

Tomato Sauce

One of our most praised recipes. Use vegetable broth or water to thin it to the right consistency for spaghetti, or use it "as is" for dishes like pizza.

Fresh tomatoes are wonderful, of course, but if they aren't in season, use canned. (Check the label to avoid added salt and sugar.)

$^1/_2$ onion, chopped

1 clove garlic

2 tablespoons olive oil

1 small carrot, grated

2 tablespoons green pepper, chopped

1 bay leaf

$^1/_2$ teaspoon oregano

$^1/_2$ teaspoon thyme

1 teaspoon basil

2 tablespoons fresh parsley, chopped

2 cups tomatoes, coarsely chopped

1 6-ounce can tomato paste

$^1/_4$ teaspoon honey

1 teaspoon salt

$^1/_8$ teaspoon pepper

▼ *Makes about 3 cups*

Sauté onion and garlic clove in oil until onion is soft. Crush garlic with a fork.

Add carrot, green pepper, bay leaf, and herbs. Stir well, then add the tomatoes, tomato paste, honey, salt, and pepper. Simmer 15 minutes. Remove the bay leaf.

❧ *Variations*

Mexican Sauce: When onion is nearly done, stir in 1 teaspoon cumin and 1 teaspoon chili powder, or to taste.

Italian Sauce: Add a pinch of fennel. Increase oregano to 1 teaspoon.

Quick Spicy Tomato Sauce*

1 tablespoon olive oil

1/2 cup shallot or red onion, chopped

2 cloves garlic

1 tablespoon coriander powder

1 teaspoon cumin

1/4 teaspoon turmeric

1/2 teaspoon salt

3 cups tomatoes, chopped

▼ *Makes 2 cups*

In oil, sauté shallot or onion with whole garlic cloves until soft. Add spices and continue cooking and stirring for a minute or so, until spices are fragrant and onion begins to brown. Stir in the tomatoes, cover, and cook gently at least until tomatoes have turned to liquid. Force through food mill or sieve.

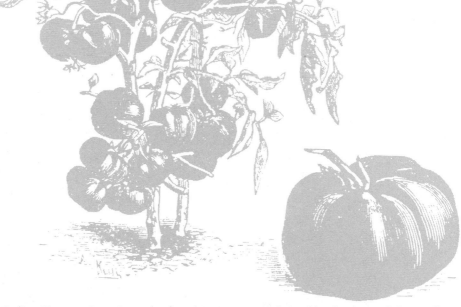

---

* Another nice "Italian Tomato Sauce" can be found in *Moosewood Cookbook (Revised)* by Mollie Katzen, published by Ten Speed Press.

WHEAT-FREE RECIPES

*Wheat-Free Pie Crust**

1 cup brown rice flour

1 cup oat flour

$^1/_4$ teaspoon sea salt

2 tablespoons sesame oil

$^2/_3$–$^3/_4$ cup water

▼ *Makes 1 pie crust*

Lightly roast the flours in a skillet, stirring to toast but not to brown. Combine all ingredients in a bowl and mix. Press mixture into oiled pie dish, spreading from center to edges to make a thin crust. Prebake for 10–15 minutes at 350°F; remove and cool before adding pie filling. This recipe can also be used with whole wheat pastry flour and chopped walnuts.

---

* A variation from *The Self-Healing Cookbook* by Kristina Turner, published by Earthtones Press.

*The Universal Cracker Recipe**

Many health food stores offer specialty flours: corn, barley, millet, buckwheat, oat, lima bean, garbanzo bean, tapioca, potato flour, rice, and so on. You can also make your own using a hand mill or a small electric nut and seed grinder, available at health food stores. To make crackers, experiment with the following recipe until you get the consistency and taste you want. You'll be surprised how easy it is, and you avoid the problems of yeast, sugar, additives, preservatives, etc.

1 cup flour

$^1/_2$ teaspoon baking soda (optional)

$^3/_4$ cup liquid (water, broth, or milk)

2 teaspoons oil

seasoning as you wish: garlic, herbs, seeds, nuts, or
   grated vegetables

▼ *Serves 6*

Combine flour and baking soda. Blend in liquid. Add oil and seasonings. Pour onto lightly oiled cookie sheet. Bake at 375°F for 5–10 minutes. Flip and bake 3 more minutes.

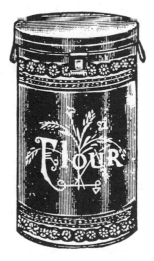

* From *Dr. Braly's Food Allergy and Nutrition Revolution* by James Braly, M.D., Kaets Publishing.

MILK/EGG-FREE RECIPES

Tofu Sour Cream and *Tofu Mayonnaises*, from the *The New Laurel's Kitchen*, are milk- and egg-free recipes for those with allergies. They are also lower in fat for people who like creamy sour cream or mayonnaise but who are watching their waistlines or cholesterol levels.

Tofu Sour Cream

This makes a tasty substitute for plain sour cream. You won't need the water with soft tofu, but with firm tofu you probably will.

> $1/4$ cup lemon juice
>
> 2 tablespoons oil
>
> 1 tablespoon light miso
>
> $1/4$ teaspoon mustard
>
> 2 tablespoons water (if using firm tofu)
>
> 1 tablespoon shoyu (or other flavoring)
>
> $1^1/2$ pounds tofu

▼ *Makes $1^1/2$ cups*

Blender: Place all ingredients except tofu in blender. Add tofu bit by bit, blending smooth with each addition. If the mixture stops moving, turn off blender and stir, then blend again. Add tofu and repeat until all is included.

Processor: Put it all in and process until creamy smooth.

Tofu Mayonnaises

Follow the directions for Tofu Sour Cream, *using the ingredients listed.*

❧ Russian

1 tablespoon white miso

1 tablespoon prepared mustard

2 tablespoons oil

3 tablespoons cider vinegar

dash pepper

pinch chili powder

1/2 teaspoon dill weed

1/8 teaspoon paprika

1/2 pound tofu

❧ Oriental

1 tablespoon shoyu or dark miso

3 tablespoons rice vinegar

white part of 2 green onions, minced

2 teaspoons ginger, minced

2 tablespoons oil

sliver fresh garlic, minced

1/2 pound tofu

❧ French Onion

2 tablespoons oil sautéed with:

1/2 small onion, minced

1 clove garlic

1/2 small carrot, grated

pinch chili powder

1/8 teaspoon paprika

2 tablespoons cider vinegar

1/8 teaspoon black pepper

1/2 pound tofu

▼ *Each recipe makes about 1 1/2 cups*

More Tofu: A couple of good tofu salads are "Eggless Egg Salad" in *The Enchanted Broccoli Forest (Revised)* by Mollie Katzen, published by Ten Speed Press, and "Marinated Tofu Salad" from *The Airola Diet and Cookbook* by Paavo Airola, published by Health Plus Publishers.

❈ ❈ ❈

For the highly vitalizing raw-food diet, seed cheeses and yogurt can provide very important nutrition. It does take some artful preparation, however, to make them right. Here are recipes from *The Hippocrates Diet and Health Program* (Avery Publishing Group) by Ann Wigmore. First make:

Rejuvelac

¹/₂ cup soft summer wheatberries
   (24-hour sprouted are best)
spring or filtered water

Grind wheatberries and put ¹/₄ cup each in 2 large jars. Fill jars almost to top with water and cover with cheesecloth and an elastic band. Allow the mixture to sit for 3 days. On the fourth day, pour off Rejuvelac, straining out berries and sediment. Store unused Rejuvelac in the refrigerator. It will keep several days. Start a new batch twice a week.

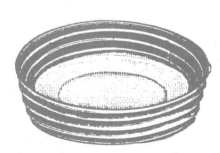
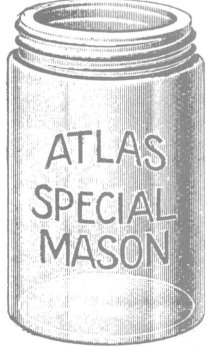

Seed Cheese

1¹/₂ cups hulled, raw sunflower seeds

¹/₂ cup hulled, raw sesame seeds

1 cup Rejuvelac or spring or filtered water

▼ *Makes about 2¹/₂ cups*

Soak seeds 8 hours and sprout for 8 hours. After this time, pour Rejuvelac into a blender. Blend at high speed, slowly adding seeds until all are blended to a smooth paste (approximately 4 minutes). Pour the mixture into a glass jar, cover with a cloth or towel, and set aside for 4–8 hours. If Rejuvelac is not available, use water and let mixture sit 2 extra hours. Or, save ¹/₄ cup from a previous cheese culture and mix it with the new batch. After the 4–8 hours have elapsed, pour off the whey by inserting a wooden spoon down one side of the jar to form a tunnel and spilling the liquid into the sink. Store it tightly covered in the refrigerator. Refrigerated, the cheese will last 5 days.

Seed Yogurt

1¹/₂ cups hulled, raw sunflower seeds

¹/₂ cup hulled, raw sesame seeds

2 cups Rejuvelac or spring or filtered water

▼ *Makes about 4 cups*

Follow the same procedure as for *Seed Cheese* (previous recipe), only set mixture aside for no more than 6 hours. Stir and refrigerate.

Bean Spreads (or Dip)

You can make bean spreads and dips with a variety of beans—garbanzos, white beans, split peas, black-eyed peas, pinto, kidney, or black beans—and a wide array of herbs, spices, and accompanying vegetables.

❧ Basics:

2 cups cooked beans,* mashed

1 tablespoon oil

1 small lemon, juiced

1 clove garlic, pressed

$1/2$ onion, chopped

cumin to taste

salt to taste

❧ Herbs and Seasoning Choices:

green pepper or chili pepper, chopped

parsley, chopped fine

green onions, chopped

$1/2$ teaspoon cumin

$1/2$–1 teaspoon chili powder

1 teaspoon basil

$1/2$ teaspoon oregano

$1/2$ teaspoon coriander

$1/4$ teaspoon thyme

1 teaspoon mustard

1–2 tablespoons red wine vinegar

1–2 tablespoons sesame tahini

▼ Makes 2 cups

Mash or blend beans with oil, lemon, garlic, and onion, then add cumin and salt and 2–3 other herbs and seasonings selected from the list of choices. Add any other ingredients of choice. To make a dip, add a little more water, lemon juice, and oil. You can use these spreads in sandwiches, or serve with crackers and vegetable sticks; celery and cucumber are good choices. In a sandwich with sliced tomato and sprouts or lettuce, these spreads provide a nutritious meal.

---

* See earlier discussion on cooking beans, pp. 41–42

BUTTER-FREE SPREADS

Here are two tasty, lowfat, butter-free, and spreadable vegetable butters by Kristina Turner in *The Self-Healing Cookbook*, published by Earthtones Press.

Sweet Carrot Butter

Sweet, creamy, and super as a spread on whole wheat toast, rice cakes, or even waffles...

4 cups carrots, sliced

$^1/_2$ cup water

pinch of sea salt

1 heaping tablespoon kudzu, dissolved in
   2 tablespoons water

1–2 tablespoons sesame tahini

▼ *Makes 1 small bowl*

Slice carrots in 1-inch chunks and place in pressure cooker with water and salt. Bring to pressure, turn down, and simmer 10 minutes. (If you don't have a pressure cooker, steam 20 minutes.) Purée carrots in blender, with $^1/_2$ cup liquid from pressure-cooking or steaming. Dissolve kudzu in cool water, mix with carrot purée, and reheat. Stir until it bubbles (kudzu must be heated thoroughly to thicken). For buttery flavor, stir in sesame tahini.

Sesame Squash Butter

Carrot butter was my #1 favorite until I invented this!

> 1 cup mashed, cooked buttercup or butternut squash
>
> 3 tablespoons sesame seeds*
>
> 1 teaspoon mellow white or chick-pea miso
>
> dash of cinnamon
>
> water

▼ *Makes 1 small bowl*

Steam, bake, or pressure-cook the squash, then mash. Roast sesame seeds by stirring in a skillet over medium heat until they smell toasty and crumble easily between thumb and forefinger. Grind into a butter in the blender or suribachi. Mix in squash, miso, and cinnamon, and add just enough water to make a creamy spread.

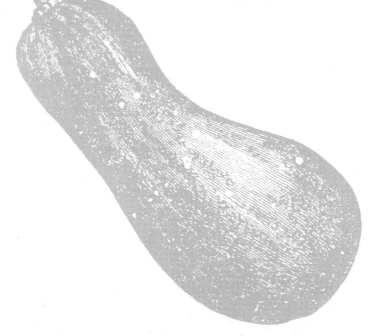

---

* Fresh roasted and ground sesame seeds add a special taste and aroma. In a rush? Substitute tahini.

QUINOA RECIPES

Due to special requests, we have included a few additional quinoa recipes. This light and nutritious whole grain contains more optimal levels of the eight essential amino acids than most other vegetable sources, making it a more complete protein. Most people find quinoa a very tasty and less congestive substitute for the more common grains, such as wheat, rice, and oats.

Mexican Quinoa with Spinach

1¹/₂ tablespoons canola oil

1 medium onion, diced

2 cloves garlic, minced

1 jalapeño pepper, minced

1 teaspoon ground cumin

1 teaspoon ground coriander

1 cup quinoa

1 bell pepper, seeded and diced

2 cups water or vegetable stock

sea salt to taste

2 cups fresh spinach, chopped

2 tablespoons fresh parsley, minced

▼ *Serves 4–6*

In a large saucepan, heat the oil and sauté the onion, garlic, and jalapeño pepper with the cumin and coriander, until onion is translucent and garlic slightly golden. Add quinoa, bell pepper, water, and salt; cover and simmer for 10 minutes. Add spinach, cover and simmer 5 to 10 more minutes, or until all liquid is absorbed. Adjust seasoning, stir in parsley, and serve.

Colorful Quinoa Salad with Raspberry Yogurt Dressing

2 medium tomatoes, cut into $1/4$-inch cubes

1 cup endive, sliced into $1/4$-inch slices

$1/2$ green pepper, seeded and diced

2 cups cooked quinoa

1 tablespoon parsley, minced

$1/4$ cup raisins

4 scallions, finely sliced

▼ *Serves 4–6*

Combine all ingredients in a large bowl.

Raspberry Yogurt Dressing

$1/2$ cup olive or canola oil

3 tablespoons raspberry vinegar

$1/2$ cup low-fat yogurt or goat yogurt

$1/2$ teaspoon honey

$1/2$ teaspoon mustard

▼ *Makes 1 cup*

Mix all ingredients in a bowl or a blender and pour over salad.

Victoria's Quinoa Cake
with Lemon Sauce

1 cup quinoa	1 cup rice syrup
³/₄ cup couscous	¹/₂ cup almonds, chopped
³/₄ cup raisins	1 teaspoon vanilla
3 cups apple juice	juice of 2 small lemons
3 cups water	zest of 2 small lemons
¹/₄ teaspoon sea salt	1 tablespoon corn oil

▼ *Makes 1 cake*

Preheat oven to 350°F.

Place quinoa, couscous, and raisins in a heavy-bottomed saucepan with the apple juice, water and salt. Bring to a boil, cover, and simmer for 20 minutes or until all liquid is absorbed. Add rice syrup, chopped almonds, vanilla, lemon juice, and lemon zest.

Oil a springform pan with the corn oil and pour mixture into it, pressing well. Bake at 350°F for 30–40 minutes. Allow to cool and unmold. Serve as a breakfast cake with orange marmalade or as a dessert with *Lemon Sauce*.

Lemon Sauce

¹/₂ cup lemon juice

2 tablespoons rice syrup

1 tablespoon sake

1 teaspoon arrowroot

▼ *Makes 1 cup*

Place all indredients in a saucepan. Bring to a boil, lower heat, and simmer, stirring constantly until sauce thickens. Transfer to a bowl and allow to cool before serving.

SPECIAL SNACKS FOR KIDS
(AND THEIR FOLKS)

There are so many poor-quality snacks marketed to kids—products that contain sugar, refined flour, preservatives, and dangerous artificial coloring—that I want to include a few recipes for healthy treats that children will like. Some of the recipes in this book may not be acceptable to many kids' usual tastes; however, the majority probably will. Some of the pastas and most breakfasts, burgers, and dips should go over quite well. Basic grain dishes, the fruit kanten, the sunshine bars, and the cookie recipes will likely be a hit. Any of the spicier recipes can also be toned down for family meals as well.

Other healthy snacks appreciated by children include: popcorn, granola, and dried fruits. However, minimize the use of dried fruits, as they can be constipating. Soaking dried fruits overnight allows them to be hydrated and often more tasty.

Kids and most anyone will love "natural" french fries, or baked fries. Cut potatoes into strips. Place on pan and bake for 10–15 minutes at 350°F until golden brown (bake with a little olive oil and salt or garlic salt and cayenne for more spicy baked "fries"). There are many fatty or sugary meals and snacks that we can make in healthier ways. Have fun in the kitchen and let your children play and create with you; they'll love it.

Frozen Juice Pops

For homemade popsicles, start with bottled, nonsugared, naturally pressed juices. Your choices of juice include: orange, papaya, orange-papaya mix, tropical punch (very tasty), apple or an apple mix such as apple boysenberry, grape, etc.

Some juices, such as grape, will taste better diluted with a little water; in general, to lessen sweetness, add some water to the juice.

Pour juice into popsicle containers and freeze. There are many new containers available in various shapes. Ice cube trays can also work; the shape is just harder to eat.

A great summer treat!

Dr. Elson's Nice Cream

Frozen desserts made of fresh fruit can only be made in certain types of juicers or food processors: machines that push out everything that goes in. Freeze peeled bananas, then push whole bananas through the juicer; they will come out as creamy banana "nice cream," a real taste treat. Carob powder, carob chips, coconut pieces, or walnuts can also be run through with the bananas for a "nice cream" variation.

Fresh frozen peaches, strawberries (trimmed), or other berries can also be used straight or mixed with bananas. I have even thrown in some frozen kiwis—peeled first, of course.

Yogurt Freezes

Many fruits also work well for these frozen treats. Either mash fruit and add yogurt, or purée fruit in the blender with a little honey or pure maple syrup. Add splash of water (or lemon juice for a tangy taste); then add plain regular, lowfat, or nonfat yogurt and blend again. You can add chopped walnuts or almonds, coconut flakes, carob powder, or natural flavorings for variation. Pour mixture into freezable cups or scoop into popsicle containers

Some sample yogurt freezes include:

- **Banana Yogurt Freeze**—2 ripe bananas, ½ teaspoon honey or maple syrup, ½ teaspoon lemon juice; and 1 cup yogurt. For carob or cocoa banana, mix in 2 tablespoons carob powder or 1 tablespoon pure cocoa.

- **Banana-Papaya**—1 medium banana with ¼–½ fresh papaya, ½ teaspoon lemon juice and 1 cup yogurt.

- **Apple**—1 cup fresh apple without skin or 1 cup applesauce, 2 teaspoons honey, a pinch of cinnamon, and 1 cup yogurt.

- **Strawberry**—1½ cups strawberries, 1 tablespoon honey, a splash of water, and 1 cup yogurt.

- **Other berries** or fruits, such as peaches or nectarines, can also be used. Blend 1–2 cups fresh or fresh frozen fruits with 1 tablespoon honey and 1 cup plain yogurt.

Nut Milks

Milk-free, nutrient-rich beverage treats can be made in a blender with a variety of nuts, water, and a touch of maple syrup and sea salt. You can use almonds, Brazil nuts, cashews, or coconut.

> $^1/_4$–$^1/_2$ cup nuts, preferably unsalted, raw whole nuts,
> or fresh coconut pieces (chopped or broken pieces
> of nuts or shredded coconut can also be used)
>
> $^3/_4$–$1^1/_2$ cups purified water
>
> 1–2 teaspoons pure maple syrup
>
> 1–2 pinches sea salt

▼ *Makes 1–2 cups*

Put nuts in blender or food processor, mash to pulp, then cover with half of the water. Blend about 30 seconds, adding half of the maple syrup and salt. Pour nut milk through strainer into bowl and transfer to a storage jar. Place nuts back into blender and repeat blending with the remaining water, maple syrup, and salt. You may vary the proportions according to taste. Again strain out the liquid nut milk. Refrigerate and serve as a drink or on cereal. Lasts several days, refrigerated (use pure coconut milk within 24 hours). The leftover nut pulp can be used in cooking, such as in grain/vegetable dishes, or in baking.

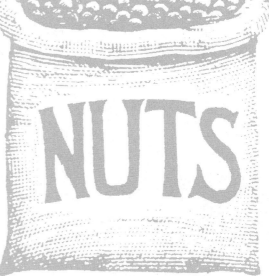

Halvah

This is a rich treat, high in protein, oil, and nutrients.

1 cup ground sesame seeds or
    1 cup raw tahini (sesame
    seed butter)
3–4 teaspoons honey (hard-
    ened, crystalline works best)

$^1/_4$ cup raisins (optional)
2–3 tablespoons shredded
    coconut (optional)

▼ *Makes 15–20 pieces*

Mash ingredients together in a small bowl and roll into balls or make into small bars. Roll on shredded coconut if desired. Can mix in 1–2 teaspoons of carob for carob halvah. Can also mash in banana for a tahini-banana mix that is very tasty.

*Tahini Candy**

$^1/_4$ cup almonds
$^1/_2$ cup tahini
4 tablespoons maple syrup

$^1/_4$ teaspoon almond extract
1 tablespoon carob flour
$^1/_4$ cup grated coconut

▼ *Serves 4*

Preheat oven to 425°F. Spread the almonds on a baking sheet and roast in the oven for 5 minutes. In a small mixing bowl, blend the tahini, maple syrup, and almond extract, beating vigorously for 3 minutes until a stiff ball forms and the oil begins to separate; stir in the carob flour. As the mixture stiffens, press the dough against the sides of the bowl with a spoon to expel the oil, then pour off. Allow the dough to sit for 1–2 minutes. Remove the almonds from the oven. Press and drain the dough again and place in a napkin or paper towel; squeeze to absorb excess oil. Chop the almonds and add to the mixture. Place the mixture on a piece of wax paper (so it won't stick to the chopping board) and roll into a cylinder shape. Slice the roll into bite-sized pieces and cover with grated coconut.

---

* This recipe is offered by Annemarie Colbin from *The Book of Whole Meals* (page 208), published by Ballantine Books.

Fruit Bars

$^1/_2$ cup honey

1 cup rolled oats

$^1/_2$ cup raisins

$^1/_2$ cup sunflower seeds

$^1/_4$ cup chopped dates or dried apricots

▼ *Makes 10–12 bars*

Heat honey in saucepan and stir in other ingredients. Pour into pan and let dry. Cut into bars and refrigerate or serve.

Puffed Rice Balls

1 cup unsalted peanuts

10 rice cakes, or equivalent amount of rice cereal

1 teaspoon vanilla extract

pinch of salt

$^1/_2$ cup raisins

$^1/_2$ cup rice syrup

▼ *Makes 10 rice balls*

Roast peanuts in oven or pan until golden and set aside. Crumble rice cakes with your hands and set aside. Place vanilla, salt, raisins and rice syrup into a frying pan and cook for 2 to 3 minutes. Add crumbled rice cakes and peanuts and mix thoroughly. Transfer rice cake mixture to a plate, slightly oil your hands, and form rice mixture into balls. Do not press too hard—and work quickly before the mixture becomes cold. Allow balls to become cold before serving or storing in a sealed container.

Almond Cookies

1½ cups almonds

½ cup rice syrup

¼ teaspoon sea salt

½ cup unbleached flour or whole wheat pastry flour

¼ cup sugar-free raspberry jam

▼ *Makes about 25 cookies*

In a food processor, grind almonds until you obtain a powder. Add two tablespoons water and the rice syrup, salt, and flour. Process until you obtain a dough-like consistency, adding more water if necessary. Preheat oven to 350°F, oil a cookie sheet, and transfer cookie mixture onto sheet using a tablespoon. Flatten with back of spoon, or using your moistened hands, give cookies the shape that you want. They should be about ¼-inch thick. Make a little dent in the center of the cookie and place some raspberry jam into it. Bake for about 15 minutes. Remove from oven and allow to cool on a rack.

Tofu Nut Spread

1 cup tofu

1 tablespoon pitted chopped soft dates, such as Medjools

2 tablespoons walnuts, chopped

▼ *Serves 4–6*

Roast walnuts in oven or skillet. Let cool. Blend tofu with dates and walnuts.

Use as a sandwich spread with jelly, instead of peanut butter, or try stuffing pitted dates with it as a treat.

PART II

SEASONAL

MENU

PLANS

AND

RECIPES

"Cauliflower is nothing but cabbage with a college education."

MARK TWAIN

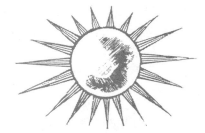

Our Ideal Diet menu plans consist of four 4-day rotation diets, one for each season. This diet/eating plan may require some adaptation from our usual way of eating. For many people, however, it may be a more radical shift, because it essentially excludes already prepared foods, such as pizza or sandwiches. Others will feel limited because they are used to more foods per meal, more variety, and especially the commonly consumed protein-starch meals, which I find the most challenging change to make in my own diet. However, this diet can be highly therapeutic for a variety of digestive problems and other health concerns. It is also very helpful in normalizing weight and minimizing food reactions or allergies in the average person. Those who have usually eaten a variety of foods and who are healthy with good digestive function will probably not need to follow strict food combining or a strict rotation diet. It is wise, though, to continue to eat simply of a variety of foods and to avoid the daily eating of specific foods, especially commonly allergenic ones such as milk, eggs, wheat, corn, soy, tomatoes, and oats.

With my guidance, Eleonora has put together these seasonal menu plans and many delicious, yet simple, recipes. Even so, our suggestions may not all be to the liking of everyone. There are, of course, many other possibilities; feel free to adapt them to feed your heart, mind, soul, and your body. Creativity is an important part of nutrition. We offer the sample menu plans and recipes primarily to educate and inspire you to follow the principles of simple, regular, wholesome meals combined so as to best promote digestion and utilization.

With the common American eight-to-five lifestyle, it may be difficult to eat our main meal at lunchtime. Our business schedule does not allow us a 1:00–4:00 P.M. break for lunch and siesta time as in many other countries. Because of this reality, some of the menu plans can allow switches between lunch and dinner; yet they are still noted as the main meal at midday because this we believe is best nutritionally. For example, on Day 3 of Spring, the fish lunch would need to be prepared the night before and taken to work. If this is not practical, the couscous dish can be eaten at lunch and the fish and vegetables prepared fresh for dinner.

I am very supportive of vegetarianism, yet I realize that most people in our culture and the world do not choose to eat this way. To be realistic and also supportive of the omnivorous diet, some of the meals in the menu plans contain fish and poultry; I have included no red meats. I believe that if we keep our priorities and food groups in the right perspective, an omnivorous diet can be equal to or healthier than a vegetarian one. Besides being easier to follow, an omnivorous diet can more readily provide all essential nutrients. In general, our menu plans and recipes are low in milk products and eggs—foods that are best eaten only moderately by most adults.

It is more common now for both vegetarians and omnivores to find a balance that combines many of the wholesome foods of the strict vegetarian with the nourishing water animals, both fresh water and ocean fish. The quality of usable protein in fish is excellent, the nutrient content is high and the digestability is very good for most people. I have termed this diet "pescoveganism"—fish and strict vegetarianism—and it is the main diet I have followed for many years.

Following the sample menus and recipes are seasonal food lists. These seasonal foods come primarily from the vegetable kingdom. Most animal foods are available year-round, and in many parts of the world, with modern technology and improved storage, a lot of fruits and vegetables can be found outside their season. If we can consume about 50–75 percent of our foods as fresh and seasonal—that is, near the area where they are grown and at the time when they are naturally harvested—that will be a good beginning.

The seasonal food lists should help you with shopping and food awareness. These lists are from *The Seasonal Food Guide* poster and booklet, also published by Celestial Arts. Our menu plans and recipes are not taken exclusively from these seasonal food lists; that expectation is unrealistic in today's world. Many foods, such as the grains, legumes, nuts, and seeds, store relatively well and are used commonly throughout the year by most people. Mainly, it is the fruits and vegetables that should bring out our seasonal awareness, and our recipes will give the suggestion that we are shopping for fresh, local produce as we hope you will. Many of our recipes can cross over seasonally, depending on the climate in which you live; and some of the recipes reprinted from other books, which often provide a combination of foods, may be used in other seasons if you wish.

CHAPTER 5
SPRING

Spring is a time of purification, healing, and rejuvenation. Nature is in her birth cycle. It is the most harmonious time of the year for fasting and cleansing the body and mind. In nature, the greens are growing freely, and these chlorophyll-rich foods are the body's best detoxifiers. In many climates, citrus and other fruits are available for cleansing as well. I usually do a ten-day *Master Cleanser* fast at the beginning of spring. (See Chapter 10 on Detoxification for a review of this important healing process.)

As spring progresses, the amount of fresh fruits and vegetables in the diet should tend to increase in proportion to other foods, such as whole grains, legumes, and the richer protein-fat foods that are consumed more in the colder, winter months. Fresh, sprouted seeds and beans are a nutritional addition to the spring menu.

Spring is a great season to reevaluate your health program and possibly create a new one, incorporating whatever changes seem necessary. Stretching exercises to enhance flexibility and openness to change are very valuable along with a good aerobic activity program for optimum health. Your body is truly ready for cleaning out the past (issues and toxins) and planting new seeds for growth and fruition within this next year's cycle.

Begin each day with two glasses of purified water (one with half a fresh squeezed lemon) and some stretching exercises. Write and repeat a few affirmations that support your goals and your will to achieve desired results. Make a schedule for your eating, exercise, and other activities. Eat plenty of the wonderful fresh fruits and vegetables available to you, as well as sprouted seeds, legumes, and nuts in your salads and other dishes. Think positively and be open to messages from within and without.

❀ SPRING MENU PLAN ❀

❂ DAY 1 ❂

Morning: One or two oranges

Breakfast: Cream of wheat or rye, plain or with a small amount of honey and oil or butter

Snack: One handful of soaked almonds

Lunch: *Pasta with Garbanzos*
Salad of mixed lettuces and spring greens (cilantro, watercress, miner's lettuce, dandelion, sorrel) and sliced red radish with *Avocado Dressing*

Snack: Glass of orange juice or whole wheat crackers

Dinner: *Puréed Carrot Soup* (with lemon, miso, and dill)
Steamed artichokes with *Tofunaise*

Snack: Herbal tea with honey

❂ DAY 2 ❂

Morning: Grapefruit

Breakfast: Cream of rice or puffed rice with yogurt or soymilk

Snack: Handful of raw or roasted pumpkin seeds

Lunch: Breast of chicken with *Tomato-Caper Sauce*
Spinach salad with *Miso-Tahini Dressing*

Snack: Rice cakes

Dinner: *Vegetable Minestrone* (with rice)
Pesto Sauce

Snack: Rice or soy ice cream (such as Rice Dream or Ice Bean)

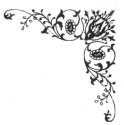

❧ DAY 3 ❧

Morning: One or two apples

Breakfast: Oatmeal cooked in water with raisins

Snack: One handful of sunflower seeds

Lunch: Broiled fresh fish (halibut, sea bass, or swordfish)
Oven roasted potatoes with rosemary
Salad of mixed greens with vinaigrette of olive oil,
balsamic vinegar, garlic, mustard, and sea salt

Snack: Carrot and celery sticks, or granola

Dinner: *Couscous Salad*
Steamed asparagus

Snack: Baked apple with raisins

❧ DAY 4 ❧

Morning: Strawberries

Breakfast: Corn puffs or flakes with soymilk

Snack: Handful of soaked filberts (hazelnuts)

Lunch: *Polenta with Tomato-Lentil Sauce*
Grated parmesan cheese (optional)
Small green salad with vinaigrette

Snack: Raw carrot and celery sticks

Dinner: *Watercress Bisque*
Sweet and Sour Tempeh or Tofu

Snack: *Strawberry-Rhubarb Pudding*

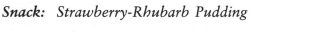

NOTE: Spring Menu Plan recipes in italics follow in the order listed.

Pasta with Garbanzos

1$\frac{1}{2}$ cups whole wheat spirals or bows

4 cups cooked or sprouted garbanzo beans

1 teaspoon thyme

1 teaspoon marjoram

1 clove garlic, minced

3 tablespoons extra virgin olive oil, or to taste

$\frac{1}{8}$ teaspoon cayenne pepper

$\frac{1}{2}$ tablespoon sea salt, or tamari

❀ *Serves 6*

Cook pasta in water and salt. Drain and combine with garbanzos, herbs, and garlic. Season with olive oil, cayenne, sea salt, or tamari. Serve hot or cold. For a whole meal, you can also add some fresh veggies and a splash of rice vinegar.

Avocado Dressing

2 medium avocados

1 lemon, juiced

1 teaspoon salt to taste

$\frac{1}{2}$ cup water

$\frac{1}{8}$ teaspoon cayenne pepper

1 clove garlic

❀ *Makes 1$\frac{1}{2}$ cups*

Blend all ingredients well and toss with salad.

Puréed Carrot Soup

7 cups water

12 medium-sized carrots, cut into pieces

$1/4$ lemon with peel

2 tablespoons light miso or to taste

2 tablespoons fresh dill

❀ *Serves 6*

Bring water to a boil. Add carrots and lemon. Cover and simmer until carrots are tender, about 10 to 20 minutes. Remove lemon and discard. Purée in blender or food processor with miso, and garnish with fresh dill. (A puréed carrot soup using carrots, onion, garlic, and celery with a squeeze of fresh ginger is a spicier autumn choice. Topped with some *Sesame Salt* [see page 58], this variation is very tasty.)

Tofunaise

6–8 ounces tofu

1 tablespoon brown rice vinegar

$1/2$ teaspoon salt or to taste

$1/2$ teaspoon ground coriander

1 teaspoon Dijon mustard (optional)

1 tablespoon olive oil

❀ *Makes $1^1/2$ cups*

Blend all ingredients.

Tomato-Caper Sauce

---

1 tablespoon olive oil

1 clove garlic

1 chili pepper

1 28-ounce can peeled tomatoes, or 1 pound fresh, peeled tomatoes

1/4 cup chopped black olives

2 tablespoons capers

sea salt to taste

❁ *Makes 4 cups*

Heat oil over medium flame and sauté garlic and chili pepper until garlic is slightly golden. Remove chili from oil and add tomatoes. Simmer with lid ajar for about 20 minutes. Add olives and capers and simmer 5 more minutes. Season to taste. Serve over baked breasts of chicken or over pasta or fish, such as snapper or cod.

Miso-Tahini Dressing

---

1 tablespoon light miso

3 tablespoons toasted sesame tahini

1 tablespoon brown rice vinegar

1/4 teaspoon rice malt or honey

3 tablespoons water

❁ *Makes 1 cup*

Blend all ingredients well. For a thinner consistency, add more water.

Vegetable Minestrone

1$\frac{1}{2}$ quarts water

1 strip kombu sea vegetable (optional)

3 shiitake stems (optional)

1$\frac{1}{2}$ cups cooked brown rice

1 tablespoon fresh or $\frac{1}{2}$ tablespoon dried thyme

1 tablespoon fresh or $\frac{1}{2}$ tablespoon dried marjoram

2 leeks, cut into $\frac{1}{2}$-inch pieces

1 potato, cut into cubes

2 stalks celery, chopped

1 cup shredded cabbage

3 small carrots, cut into pieces

1 cup broccoli florets

1 cup sweet peas

sea salt to taste

❀ *Serves 6*

Bring water, kombu, shiitake stems, and herbs (if using dried) to a boil, and simmer for 10 minutes. Add leeks, potato, celery, cabbage, and carrots, and simmer 15 minutes longer. Then add broccoli florets, sweet peas, and herbs (if using fresh), and simmer another 10 minutes. Remove kombu and shiitake stems, season to taste, and serve.

If using leftover cooked rice, simmer vegetables in same order, and add 1$\frac{1}{2}$ cups of rice at the end. Cooking time is approximately 25–30 minutes. If serving with *Pesto Sauce* (next recipe) omit thyme and marjoram.

This soup is also very good served cold with a sprinkling of olive oil.

Pesto Sauce

1 bunch fresh basil or spinach, cleaned and
   with stems removed

1 tablespoon light miso

1 clove garlic

$1/4$ cup pine nuts and/or walnuts (optional)

3 tablespoons olive oil

parsley (optional)

❀ *Makes about 1 cup*

Purée all ingredients well in a blender or food processor. Some fresh parsley can be
added to blender to deepen the green color. If too thick, dilute with a little water.
Pass at the table and add to *Vegetable Minestrone* (previous recipe). Of course, this
nondairy pesto can be used for pastas or grain/vegetable dishes if you so desire. A
more traditional (and fattening) pesto sauce will use grated Romano cheese and more
olive oil.

Couscous Salad

2 cups whole wheat couscous

4 cups boiling water

$^{1}/_{4}$ cup chopped black olives

$^{1}/_{4}$ cup capers

1 red bell pepper, cut into small pieces

1 stalk celery, cut into small pieces

2 green onions, thinly sliced

1 cup parsley, minced

$^{1}/_{4}$ cup olive oil

2 teaspoons ume vinegar (or 1 tablespoon lemon juice
with $^{1}/_{2}$ teaspoon sea salt), or to taste

$^{1}/_{4}$ teaspoon cayenne pepper

lettuce leaves

cherry tomatoes

❀ *Serves 6*

Place couscous in a bowl and pour boiling water over it. Cover and let sit for 10 minutes. Fluff with fork. Add olives, capers, vegetables, and parsley and toss with olive oil, ume vinegar, and cayenne. Serve over a bed of lettuce garnished with cherry tomatoes.

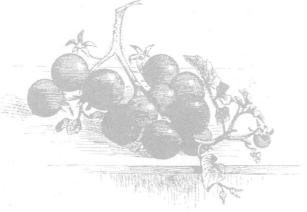

Polenta

Polenta is even better the second day. It can be baked, broiled, or grilled.

> **9 cups water or stock**
> **1 teaspoon sea salt**
> **3 cups polenta (corn grits)**

❀ *Serves 6*

Bring water and salt to a boil. Slowly add polenta while stirring constantly with a whisk until well mixed. Lower flame to minimum, cover pot, and simmer until polenta has thickened, about 20–30 minutes. Stir frequently to avoid burning. Transfer the polenta to a glass loaf pan, and let sit for 5 minutes. Cut into squares and serve with *Tomato-Lentil Sauce* (next recipe).

Tomato-Lentil Sauce

1/2 onion, finely chopped

1 carrot, finely chopped

1 stalk celery, finely chopped

1 clove garlic, minced

2 tablespoons olive oil

16 ounces fresh peeled tomatoes
   or 2 8-ounce cans

1 cup lentils

1 cup mushrooms, coarsely
   sliced

sea salt and pepper to taste

Parmesan cheese (optional)

❀ *Serves 6*

Sauté onion, carrot, celery, and garlic in oil until onions are limp and transparent. Add tomatoes and lentils and simmer 30 to 40 minutes with lid ajar. Add mushrooms, cook 5 minutes longer, and season to taste with salt and pepper. Serve over *Polenta* (previous recipe). This sauce is also excellent over pasta or whole grains. If desired, sprinkle Parmesan cheese over sauce.

Watercress Bisque

1 onion, finely chopped

1 carrot, finely chopped

1 cup dry white wine (optional)

8 cups water

2 bunches watercress (about 8 cups), coarsely
    chopped, including stems

2 tablespoons light miso, or to taste

lemon wedges to garnish

❀ *Serves 6*

Simmer onion and carrot in wine (or ½ cup water) until onion is limp and transparent. Add water and chopped watercress; cover and simmer for 20 minutes. Purée in blender or food processor with miso. Serve garnished with a lemon wedge.

Sweet and Sour Tempeh or Tofu

¹/₄ cup water

¹/₄ cup tamari

¹/₂ teaspoon ground coriander seed

1 clove garlic, minced

2 packages tempeh (1 pound) or 1 pound tofu,
   cut into 1-inch squares

¹/₄ cup arrowroot flour

peanut or rice bran oil for deep frying

❀ *Serves 6*

Mix water, tamari, coriander, and garlic. Dip tempeh or tofu cubes in mix and coat with arrowroot flour. Heat oil in a wok or skillet, and deep fry tempeh or tofu until golden. Drain well on a paper towel. For a low-fat recipe, avoid frying by omitting arrowroot and oil; marinate tofu or tempeh and bake at 350°F for 15–20 minutes. Serve with *Sweet and Sour Sauce* (next recipe).

Sweet and Sour Sauce

1¹/₂ cups water

1 cup rice syrup

4 teaspoons tamari

2 tablespoons rice vinegar

1 tablespoon tahini

¹/₂ teaspoon grated fresh ginger

1 tablespoon kudzu, diluted in
   2 tablespoons cold water

2 green onions, finely chopped

❀ *Serves 6*

Combine water, rice syrup, tamari, vinegar, tahini, and ginger and bring to a boil. Add diluted kudzu and stir until sauce thickens. Add green onions. One use for this sauce is to pour over *Sweet and Sour Tempeh or Tofu* (previous recipe).

Strawberry-Rhubarb Pudding

5 cups strawberries, sliced

2 cups rhubarb, diced

3 tablespoons maple syrup, or to taste

1 teaspoon grated lemon rind

2 tablespoons agar-agar flakes

1 tablespoon kudzu, diluted in 2 tablespoons
   cold water

❀ *Serves 6*

Bring strawberries, rhubarb, maple syrup, and lemon rind to a boil and sprinkle in agar-agar flakes. Simmer until all flakes are dissolved (about 10 minutes). Add dissolved kudzu and stir until mixture thickens. Transfer to a bowl or individual cups and refrigerate until set. Garnish with strawberry slices and a sprig of mint.

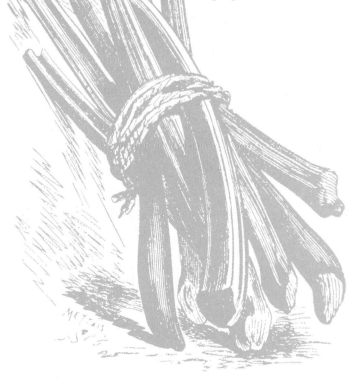

White Bean Florentine Soup

10 cups water

2 cups small white or navy beans, soaked overnight

$1/2$ cup onions, sliced

$1/2$ cup carrots, chopped

$1/2$ cup celery, chopped

1 tablespoon fresh oregano

1 tablespoon fresh basil

2 cups spinach, coarsely chopped

tamari to taste

parsley to garnish

❀ *Serves 4–6*

In a heavy-bottomed saucepan, bring water to a boil and cook beans over medium heat until they are soft and creamy, about 40 minutes. Add onion, carrots, and celery and continue to cook for 20 minutes. Add more water if soup becomes too thick. Add herbs and cook 10 more minutes. Add spinach, season to taste with tamari, and garnish with fresh parsley.

Artichoke Stew

3 tablespoons olive oil

1 small onion

$1/2$ pound small white or navy beans

8 baby artichokes

juice of 1 lemon

4 garlic cloves

sea salt to taste

pepper to taste

2 sprigs fresh thyme

4 sprigs parsley

4 cloves

2 bunches (approximately $1/2$ pound) spinach

❀ *Serves 6*

Soak beans overnight. In a heavy-bottomed saucepan, heat 1 tablespoon oil and sauté onion until translucent. Add beans, cover with water, and simmer until done, about 30–40 minutes.

Remove tough outer leaves of artichokes, and cut off tops and most of the stems. Peel remaining part of stems. Cut each artichoke in quarters, and remove the fuzzy inner part. Drizzle with some lemon juice to avoid browning.

Heat 1 tablespoon of oil in a heavy-bottomed saucepan and sauté garlic cloves until golden. Add artichoke pieces, a little salt and pepper, and the herbs, together with some of the cooking water from the beans. In another pot, rinse spinach and simmer, covered with only the water on its leaves and a little salt.

Combine all ingredients together and serve hot or cold with a drizzle of lemon juice and the remaining olive oil.

Fettuccine Primavera with Curry

3 medium carrots

1 medium onion

1 celery stick

6 thin asparagus spears

4 tablespoons olive oil

1 tablespoon mild curry powder

1 pound fettuccine

1 tablespoon pine nuts, toasted

sea salt to taste

❀ *Serves 4–6*

Finely chop carrots, onion, and celery. Slice asparagus diagonally into ½-inch pieces. In a heavy-bottomed saucepan, heat oil and sauté vegetables over medium heat for about 5 minutes. Add curry and a little water and simmer for a few more minutes. Boil fettuccine in plenty of salted water until al dente. Toss with curried vegetables and toasted pine nuts.

Brown Rice
with Peas and Fava Beans

1 cup shelled fava beans

3 cups long-grain brown rice

1 cup fresh shelled peas

4 scallions, finely sliced

1 tablespoon minced chives

1 tablespoon minced dill

3 tablespoons olive oil

juice of $1/2$ lemon

sea salt to taste

$1/4$ teaspoon cayenne (optional)

❀ *Serves 6*

Drop shelled fava beans in boiling water and cook for two minutes. Drain and remove skin. Cook rice in six cups water for 50–60 minutes, or until all liquid is absorbed. Add fava beans and peas to rice a few minutes before it is finished; cover and allow vegetables to cook with the steam of the rice. Marinate sliced scallions, dill, and chives for 10 minutes in olive oil, lemon juice, salt, and cayenne (if desired). Toss rice with marinade.

Zucchini Flowers
with Tofu Filling

12 zucchini flowers

¹/₂ cup whole wheat pastry flour

1 cup sparkling mineral water

1 cup tofu, crumbled

1 tablespoon light miso

12 Kalamata olives, pitted, or
    6 sun-dried tomatoes, soaked

peanut oil for deep frying

pinch of salt

❈ *Serves 6*

Remove pistils from zucchini flowers and soak flowers in cold water for 20 minutes or longer. The longer they are soaked, the crisper they will be.

Place flour and mineral water in freezer for 15 minutes. In a bowl, mash together tofu and miso.

Remove zucchini flowers from water and place on a paper towel to dry. When dry, put 1 teaspoon of the tofu/miso mixture and then a pitted olive or half a sun-dried tomato into the top part of each flower. Roll up and place on a plate.

Heat oil in a skillet.

Using a whisk, quickly mix together flour, mineral water, and salt. Dip each flower into the batter and deep fry until golden. Remove from oil with a slotted spoon and place on a plate with a paper towel to drain excess oil.

NOTE: For lower fat and to avoid fried foods, the zucchini flowers can be baked at 450°F for 10 minutes or until golden.

For a non-vegetarian filling, try a piece of mozzarella and half an anchovy or an equivalent amount of anchovy paste.

❀ ADDITIONAL SPRING RECIPES ❀

Complete information on the books used for these additional recipes will be noted in the Recipe Book Bibliography at the end of this section.

Lime Garlic Shrimp

from *Tropic Cooking* by Joyce LeFray Young

Lime is a perfect fruit for the diet-conscious; it adds a nice zest to many dishes, without adding any calories to speak of. Be careful not to overcook the shellfish!

2 pounds medium shrimp, cleaned, peeled,
    and deveined

1/4 cup butter or margarine (canola oil is
    a better choice)

4 cloves garlic, minced

1 cup minced green onions

1/4 cup freshly squeezed lime juice

coarsely ground black pepper

Tabasco or other hot sauce to taste

1/4 cup freshly chopped parsley

❀ *Serves 4–6*

Prepare the shrimp and set aside.

In a large sauté pan, melt the butter or margarine. Add the garlic and green onions and sauté until the onions turn bright green. Add the shrimp and lime juice. Maintain the heat and cook just briefly, until shrimp turns pink. Stir in the black pepper, hot sauce, and parsley.

Serve over fluffy rice or on toasted, buttered rolls.

Green Jade Soup

from *The Tao of Cooking* by Sally Pasley

3 dried Chinese mushrooms

4 cups vegetable stock

$1/3$ cup carrots, peeled and cut in 1-inch matchsticks

$1/4$ cup thinly sliced green onions

$1/2$ cup thinly sliced mushrooms

about 10 spinach leaves

3 tablespoons soy sauce

❀ *Serves 4*

Soak dried mushrooms in 1 cup hot water for 20–30 minutes, until soft. Drain and reserve stock. Slice in thin strips.

Bring reserved mushroom stock and vegetable stock to a boil in saucepan. Add carrots, green onions, and both kinds of mushrooms and simmer for 3 minutes. Add spinach leaves and soy sauce and cook for a few more minutes, until spinach is just wilted. Taste for seasoning.

Serve this simple, clear soup with nori rolls or tempura. You may also add thin Japanese noodles for a more filling soup.

Watercress Salad

from *The Airola Diet and Cookbook*
by Paavo Airola

1 bunch fresh watercress

$^1/_4$ pound fresh mushrooms, washed and sliced

1 cup mung bean sprouts

1 tablespoon chopped fresh parsley

1 green onion, chopped

3 tablespoons cold-pressed olive oil

1 tablespoon red wine vinegar

$^1/_8$ teaspoon sea salt

dash of cayenne pepper

❀ *Serves 4*

Wash the watercress and tear into bite-sized pieces. Combine the watercress with the sliced mushrooms, bean sprouts, parsley, and green onion. Make a dressing with the olive oil, red wine vinegar, sea salt, and cayenne and pour over the salad, or use *Pollution Solution Dressing* (next recipe).

Pollution Solution Dressing

from *The Airola Diet and Cookbook*
by Paavo Airola

This salad dressing is specially formulated to minimize the damage from environmental pollution. It contains factors that have been shown to be effective in protecting the body from the toxic effects of heavy metal poisoning, such as from lead, mercury, and cadmium, as well as minimizing the damage from X-rays and other sources of harmful environmental radiation. Can use with any salad.

1 cup mayonnaise or *Tofunaise*
  (see recipe on page 91)

1 ripe tomato, chopped

1 small dill pickle, chopped

2 tablespoons chopped onion

2 tablespoons chopped green pepper

3 cloves of garlic, minced

2 teaspoons honey

1 tablespoon plain yogurt

1 tablespoon lemon juice

1 tablespoon algin powder (sodium alginate)

1 tablespoon brewer's yeast flakes

2 teaspoons lecithin granules

1 teaspoon kelp

1/2 teaspoon sea salt

dash of cayenne pepper

❀ *Makes about 2 cups*

Combine all the ingredients and mix well. Store in the refrigerator.

Rice and Vegetable Salad

from *The Book of Whole Meals*
by Annemarie Colbin

1 carrot

1/2 bunch watercress

4 green onions

2 celery stalks

2 cups cooked brown rice

❀ *Serves 4*

Shred carrot with a potato peeler. Remove the stems from the watercress; chop green onions and celery stalks. Now combine the vegetables in a salad bowl, stir in the rice, and toss with *Creamy Parsley Dressing* (next recipe).

Creamy Parsley Dressing

from *The Book of Whole Meals* by Annemarie Colbin

2 ounccs soft tofu

2 tablespoons tahini

1/2 cup water

2 tablespoons brown rice vinegar (or lemon juice)

1/2 teaspoon sea salt, or to taste

1 handful washed parsley

❀ *Makes about 2 cups*

Place all ingredients in a blender and purée until creamy. Pour approximately 1/4 cup of the dressing on the *Rice and Vegetable Salad* (previous recipe). Toss well.

Pasta with Greens and Feta

from *Still Life With Menu* by Mollie Katzen

Here is a painless way to slip some of those ultranutritious bitter greens into your diet. You can use any combination of kale, mustard, collard, dandelion, escarole, chard, or spinach. I especially like escarole and spinach together.

6 tablespoons olive oil

4 cups chopped onion

7–8 cups (packed) mixed bitter greens, washed, dried, and coarsely chopped (I use 1 medium-sized bunch each spinach and escarole)

salt to taste

$3/4$–1 pound penne, fusilli, shells, or some comparable short, substantial pasta

$1/2$–$3/4$ pound feta cheese, crumbled

freshly grated Parmesan cheese, to taste (optional)

freshly ground black pepper

❀ *Serves 4–6*

Heat the olive oil in a deep skillet or Dutch oven. Add the onions and cook for about 10 minutes over medium heat, stirring occasionally. Meanwhile, put the pasta water up to boil.

Add chopped greens to the skillet, salt lightly, and stir until the greens begin to wilt. Cover and cook 10–15 minutes over medium-low heat.

Cook the pasta until al dente. Just as it becomes ready, add the crumbled feta cheese to the sauce. (Keep the heat on low as you add the cheese.)

When the pasta is done, scoop it out with a strainer (in however many batches it takes), hold it over its cooking water momentarily to drain, then add it directly to the potful of sauce. Mix thoroughly.

Cook the completed dish just slightly over low heat for a few minutes. Add a small amount of Parmesan, if desired, and a generous amount of freshly ground black pepper. Then serve immediately, preferably on warmed plates.

SPRING FOODS*

Fruits

Avocado
Date
Grapefruit
Jicama
Lemon
Lime
Loquat
Olive
Orange
Strawberry
Tangelo
Tangerine

Vegetables

Artichoke
Asparagus
Beets
Beet greens
Bok choy
Broccoli
Brussels
  sprouts
Cabbage
Cauliflower
Carrot
Celery
Chard
Chickweed
Chicory
Chives
Cilantro
Collard greens
Comfrey
Dandelion
  greens
Green garlic
Green onion

Green peas
Kale
Leeks
Lettuce:
  Butter
  Greenleaf
  Iceberg
  Redleaf
  Romaine
Miner's lettuce
Mint
Mushroom
Mustard
  greens
Nettle
Parsley
Radish
Rhubarb
Sorrel greens
Spinach
Sprouts
Sugar peas
Watercress

Sprouts

Grains:
  Barley
  Buckwheat
  Corn
  Rice
  Rye
  Wheat

Beans:
  Adzuki
  Garbanzo
  Lentil
  Mung

Seeds:
  Alfalfa
  Clover
  Radish
  Sunflower

Grains

Sprouted

Beans

Fava
Sprouted

---

* These are the foods that are usually available in the spring. This may vary slightly between locales. In some areas, certain foods may not be available until later spring or even summer. Of course, foods that can be dried after their harvest or that are naturally contained in a protective coating are available in most areas throughout the year. These include the whole grains, beans, seaweeds, seeds, and nuts. Although they are often eaten in the spring, they would not be classified as "Spring Foods."

For more complete information on the Seasonal Diets, see *The Seasonal Food Guide* poster from Celestial Arts, Berkeley, CA.

CHAPTER 6

SUMMER

Summer is a time of growth and activity, when nature and life are expanding. The warmth of summer requires both a lighter diet and fresher, higher-water-content foods. It's no accident that Nature provides a rainbow array of exactly that type of fruit and vegetable fare. This is an ideal season to experiment with special diets, like *Raw Foods* (see page 216), or a short fast (see page 235) as a transition to a new diet.

After the greens of spring blossom into fruit, many more succulent fruits and vegetables can be harvested to feed us in summer. Now we can consume more liquids and raw, fresh foods to balance and cool us during these hotter months. Generally a lighter diet is helpful unless you are extremely active or do intense physical labor—then you'll need to eat more to maintain your energy and weight. Try to eat your heavier meals during the cooler parts of the day, like early morning or early evening, so as not to overwork your digestive system.

For most of us, the foods higher in fats and proteins are best reduced in summer to allow the simpler fuels to run our bodies. Fresh salads with light dressings, cool soups, and meals made of grains and vegetables will keep you feeling light and energetic. Sprouted foods can be mixed in a variety of dishes. Also, juicy fruits and especially melons and berries may be eaten daily; however, try eating them alone for best digestion.

Summer is a time for more outdoor activity, and a full exercise program will invigorate you. Daily stretching, some weight work, outdoor bike riding, hiking, and swimming can provide the balance you need for a healthier body. So, keep your body moving this summer and drink more water, juices, and herbal teas to keep you hydrated, especially when you are active in the warm weather.

❂ SUMMER MENU PLAN ❂

❧ DAY ·1 ❧

Fruit: Fresh berries

Breakfast: *Breakfast Rice*, or puffed rice or rye flakes with yogurt

Snack: Soaked almonds

Lunch: Salad of mixed greens, chives, grated carrots, tomatoes, and tuna (or a mixture of bean sprouts or tofu salad for the vegetarian) with a vinaigrette of avocado or olive oil, lemon juice, Dijon mustard, herb salt, and cayenne

Snack: Peaches

Dinner: *Stuffed Bell Peppers*
Steamed Swiss chard sprinkled with roasted pumpkin seeds, minced garlic, olive oil, and soy sauce or tamari

Snack: Rice cake with apple butter, or papaya

❧ DAY 2 ❧

Fruit: Plums

Breakfast: Cream of wheat, *Crepes with Fruit*, or *Scrambled Tofu*

Snack: Wheat crackers or sprouted wheat toast with tahini

Lunch: Cold pasta salad with fava beans, fresh basil, lightly steamed asparagus tips, baby (or sliced) carrots, and black olives with garlic oil, sea salt, and cayenne, served over a bed of lettuce

Snack: Cherries

Dinner: *Chicken "en Chemise"*
Steamed artichoke with dilled tofu mayonnaise
Watercress and baby lettuces with safflower oil, balsamic vinegar, and sea salt

Snack: *Fruit Sorbet*

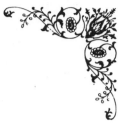

❦ DAY 3 ❦

Fruit: Oranges

Breakfast: Granola with *Fruit Kanten*

Snack: Walnuts

Lunch: Broiled halibut basted with marinade of tamari, sesame oil, garlic, fresh thyme, and fresh marjoram
Vegetable melange of lightly steamed sweet peas and carrots served with fresh arugula and a vinaigrette of olive oil, lemon or balsamic vinegar, and a pinch of sea salt

Snack: Apricots

Dinner: *Moussaka*, baby spinach with *Honey Mustard Vinaigrette*

Snack: Strawberries, blackberries, or fresh figs

❦ DAY 4 ❦

Fruit: Grapefruit

Breakfast: Corn flakes with soymilk or
Corn Bread with *Peanut-Apple Butter*

Snack: Sunflower seeds

Lunch: Fresh corn on the cob with sweet, unpasteurized butter, or lime juice
Mexican Salad Bowl

Snack: Banana

Dinner: *Baked Dill Salmon*
Green beans
Salad of Belgian Endive

Snack: Fresh berries

NOTE: Summer Menu Plan recipes in italics follow in the order listed.

Breakfast Rice

1¹/₂ cups raisins

1 tablespoon grated lemon rind

1 cinnamon stick or ¹/₂ teaspoon powder

1¹/₂ cups apple juice

5 cups leftover cooked rice

¹/₂ cup walnuts or almonds, coarsely chopped and
lightly roasted

✿ *Serves 6*

Simmer raisins, lemon rind, and cinnamon stick (or powder) in apple juice for a few minutes, until raisins are plump. Add rice, simmer a few more minutes, turn off heat, add walnuts or almonds, and let stand covered for 10 minutes or longer before serving.

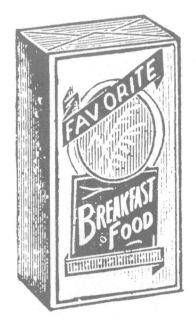

Stuffed Bell Peppers

6 bell peppers

3 tablespoons sesame oil (or water or wine)

1 clove garlic, minced

1 cup tempeh, crumbled, or 1 cup cooked beans
    (white, navy, or adzuki)

2 cups cooked leftover rice

2 green onions, finely chopped, including green part

3 tablespoons fresh cilantro, chopped, or 1 teaspoon
    coriander powder

2 tablespoons salsa (optional)

sea salt to taste

✿ *Serves 6*

Preheat oven to 400°F.

Cut tops off peppers and set aside. Scoop out seeds and white part and discard. Rinse peppers and turn over on wooden board to drain.

Heat oil (or water, or wine for lower fat) in skillet and sauté garlic and tempeh until golden brown. Add rice, green onions, cilantro, and salsa and mix well. Salt to taste and fill peppers with the mixture. Place peppers in Pyrex or other oven-proof dish, put tops back on them, and bake at 400°F for 30 minutes.

A sauce can be made to cover peppers before baking. Either top simply with 3–4 ounces of grated Monterey Jack cheese, or blend 4 ounces of tofu with 1 tablespoon tamari, 1 teaspoon of tahini, and 2–3 tablespoons of water, depending on consistency desired.

Crepes with Fruit

☙ *Batter*:

2 cups whole wheat pastry flour

¹/₄ teaspoon salt

2 tablespoons corn oil (optional)

4 cups sparkling mineral water

✿ *Serves* 6

Place flour and salt in a bowl; if using oil, work it in with your fingers until it is evenly distributed. Add mineral water slowly, stirring quickly with a whisk. Do not stir too much; the mixture should be bubbly. Use immediately.

Oil a crepe pan or a 9-inch cast-iron skillet and heat over medium flame. Pour ¹/₄ cup crepe batter into the center of the hot pan and tilt the pan quickly in all directions, so that the batter evenly covers the bottom of the pan. Cook about 5 minutes or until the edges of the crepe begin to shrink. Lift crepe with a spatula and turn over. Cook another 2 minutes. Place crepes on individual plates, spread filling over each crepe, and roll up.

NOTE: This is a light and low-fat crepe; the bubbly water takes the place of egg to make the crepes fluffy.

☙ *Filling*:

1 cup apple juice

3 cups seasonal fruit such as peaches, berries, or
    apricots

pinch of salt

2 tablespoons kudzu or arrowroot powder, diluted in
    3 tablespoons cold water or juice

Bring juice, fruit, and salt to a boil and simmer for a few minutes. Add dissolved kudzu and stir until mixture thickens.

Scrambled Tofu

Lighter than eggs, and lower in fat.

1¹/₂ pounds tofu

2 tablespoons light miso

1 tablespoon sesame oil

1 cup mushrooms, sliced

¹/₄ cup black olives, minced

2 medium tomatoes, seeded and chopped

1 teaspoon turmeric

¹/₄ teaspoon cayenne, or to taste

sea salt to taste

¹/₄ cup fresh parsley or cilantro, minced

2 green onions, thinly sliced

✲ *Serves 6*

Place tofu in a bowl with miso and mash together thoroughly. Heat oil in skillet and sauté mushrooms for a few minutes. Add tofu mixture, olives, tomatoes, and turmeric. Stir together well, cover, and simmer over low flame for 5 minutes. Season to taste with cayenne and sea salt, add parsley or cilantro and green onions, and serve. Add or substitute onion and garlic, carrot (diced or grated), and celery slices for variety. To vary flavor, try nutritional yeast, thyme or rosemary, and dill. For spicy, scrambled tofu, add ¹/₂ teaspoon curry powder to the turmeric.

Chicken "en Chemise"

6 chicken breasts

6 pieces parchment paper

1 stalk celery, minced

1 onion, minced

1 teaspoon thyme

1 teaspoon marjoram

1 teaspoon herb salt

freshly ground black pepper or cayenne pepper

6 tablespoons lemon juice

6 tablespoons dry white wine (optional)

parsley to garnish

✪ *Serves 6*

Preheat oven to 375°F.

Season chicken breasts on both sides and place on paper squares. Place celery, onion, and herbs, on the chicken; add lemon juice, pepper, and wine; and fold ends of paper upward to form a little package. Bake for 30 minutes. Before serving, garnish with fresh parsley.

NOTE: You can use a covered Pyrex baking dish to bake chicken breasts without their chemises.

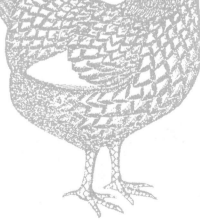

Fruit Sorbet

4 cups fresh orange juice

3 tablespoons maple syrup

2 tablespoons grated orange rind

2 cups fresh or frozen strawberries, chopped,
　　or local berries, whole

fresh mint sprigs for garnish

orange slices for garnish

✿ *Serves 6*

Blend first four ingredients together in food processor or blender. Transfer to a bowl and freeze for 2–3 hours, until solid. Break into large chunks and blend again until creamy and smooth. Return to the bowl and freeze again for about 30 minutes. Serve in individual parfait glasses with a sprig of mint and a slice of orange.

Fruit Kanten (Jelled Fruit Dessert)

7 cups apple (or other) juice

4 tablespoons agar-agar flakes

1 teaspoon vanilla extract

1 cup fresh strawberries,
　　or other seasonal fruit, sliced

3 cups granola

✿ *Serves 6*

Bring juice and agar-agar flakes to a boil and simmer covered until flakes have dissolved, about 10 minutes. Add vanilla. Arrange fruit in the bottom of a rectangular shallow glass pan and pour juice over it. Chill until set. Cut into squares and serve this natural "jello" topped with granola. This recipe can also be made in individual glass cups or parfait glasses.

Moussaka

2 large eggplants, cut in ¼-inch slices

3 tablespoons olive oil

1 large onion, sliced into crescents

2 large tomatoes, peeled, seeded, and chopped

½ cup white wine (optional)

sea salt to taste

2 cups cooked chickpeas (garbanzos)

1 tablespoon fresh oregano

3 tablespoons fresh basil

1 cup feta cheese, crumbled (optional)

✪ *Serves 6*

Preheat oven to 300°F and bake eggplant slices for about 10 minutes, or until tender enough to be pierced with a fork. Heat olive oil in a skillet and sauté onion until limp and transparent. Add tomatoes, wine, and salt. Cook uncovered for 2–3 minutes. Add chickpeas and herbs and cook a few minutes longer. Season to taste. Place one layer of eggplant slices in the bottom of a casserole dish, cover with chickpea mixture, then sprinkle feta; add another layer of eggplant, and continue until all ingredients are used. Top with feta, cover, and bake 20 minutes at 350°F. Remove cover and bake another 5 minutes.

Honey Mustard Vinaigrette

3 tablespoons grainy mustard

2 tablespoons honey

1 tablespoon tamari

1 tablespoon apple cider vinegar

5 tablespoons canola oil

✪ *Makes 1 cup*

Blend all ingredients together in a blender, or mix in a bowl using a whisk.

Corn Bread

This is a healthy, milk-free, sweet breakfast corn bread. For a richer, spicier, milkier bread, see the "Rich Jalapeño Corn Bread" recipe on page 167 in the Autumn recipes.

1 cup whole wheat pastry flour

1 cup cornmeal or corn flour

1 tablespoon baking powder (aluminum-free, if available)

$^1/_8$ teaspoon sea salt

$^1/_4$ cup sunflower seeds (optional)

$^3/_4$ cup soymilk

$^1/_4$ cup water

$^1/_4$ cup corn oil

$^1/_4$ cup pure maple syrup

$^1/_8$ teaspoon vanilla extract

✪ *Makes 1 loaf*

Preheat oven to 350°F.

Mix flour, cornmeal, baking powder, salt, and sunflower seeds in a bowl.

In a separate bowl, beat soymilk, water, corn oil, maple syrup, and vanilla together using a whisk.

Combine wet and dry ingredients. Stir a few times. Do not stir too much or the dough will become tough.

Pour into oiled loaf pan and bake at 350°F for 45 minutes to 1 hour. Check with a toothpick; when it comes out clean, the bread is done.

Peanut-Apple Butter

$^3/_4$ cup apple butter or apple sauce

$^1/_4$ cup peanut butter

✪ *Makes 1 cup*

Blend together until smooth.

Mexican Salad Bowl

3 tablespoons fresh lemon juice

2 teaspoons mustard

1 tablespoon ume vinegar (or apple cider and
   sea salt), or to taste

3 tablespoons tahini

4 tablespoons water

2 heads butter lettuce or other green lettuce, shredded

2 green onions, finely sliced

1 cucumber, grated

1 small bunch red radishes, grated

4 cups cooked black beans

2 tablespoons minced cilantro or 1 teaspoon ground
   coriander (optional)

✿ *Serves 6*

Blend lemon juice, mustard, vinegar, tahini, and water together to make the dressing.
(For a more Mexican dressing, use 3 tablespoons salsa, 1 tablespoon sesame oil, and
1/2 teaspoon salt or 1 teaspoon tamari.) Assemble all other ingredients in salad bowl
and toss with dressing.

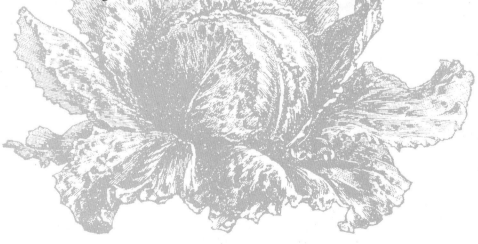

Baked Dill Salmon

2 tablespoons soy sauce

2 tablespoons lemon juice

6 salmon fillets

6 lemon slices

6 tomato slices

6 sprigs of fresh dill

✪ *Serves 6*

Preheat oven to 375°F.

    Mix together soy sauce and lemon juice, and dip salmon fillets in mixture to coat both sides. Place the fillets in a large baking dish; place a lemon slice, a tomato slice, and a sprig of dill on top and then cover with lid or foil. Bake about 20 minutes.

Salad of Belgian Endive

1 tablespoon light miso

1¹/₂ tablespoons tahini

1 tablespoon lemon juice

3 tablespoons water

1 large head butter lettuce or other green lettuce, shredded

6 endives, horizontally cut into ¹/₂-inch pieces

4 tablespoons chives, minced

✪ *Serves 6*

Blend miso, tahini, lemon juice, and water together and toss with salad, or use *Miso-Tahini Dressing* (see recipe page 92).

❧ OTHER SUMMER RECIPES ❧ FROM ELEONORA

Tofu Aspic

$1/2$ pound tofu

8 cups vegetable stock

2 tablespoons miso

$1/8$ teaspoon saffron

3 small carrots, thinly sliced on diagonal

$1/2$ cup sugar snap peas, ends removed

1 tablespoon agar-agar flakes

2 bunches chervil, minced

❃ *Serves 6*

Cut tofu into $1/2$-inch squares and boil 5 minutes in the vegetable stock. Dilute miso and saffron in $1/2$ cup water and add to vegetable stock and tofu, together with carrots and sugar snap peas. Add agar-agar flakes, cover and simmer 5 minutes, or until agar is dissolved. Add minced chervil and transfer mixture to a glass dish. Refrigerate until set. Can be served in the glass dish or unmolded onto a serving platter and surrounded by fresh watercress.

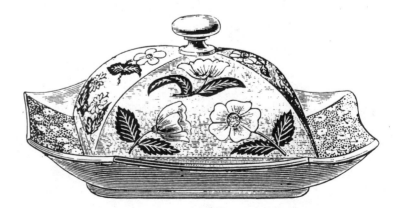

Ratatouille

1 large eggplant, cut into small cubes

3 tablespoons olive oil

sea salt and pepper to taste

10 basil leaves

¹/₂ cup pine nuts

6 medium ripe tomatoes

3 or 4 medium zucchini, cut into small cubes

1 dill sprig

1 medium onion, finely sliced

1 clove

1 cup nonfat yogurt or goat yogurt

❂ *Serves 4–6*

Soak eggplant cubes in cold water for 20 minutes. Drain and pat dry with a paper towel. Heat 2 tablespoons oil in a heavy-bottomed saucepan and sauté eggplant until soft. Season with salt and pepper. Blend basil with pine nuts and 1 tablespoon olive oil in a blender and add to eggplant.

Plunge tomatoes in boiling water for a few seconds, peel them, cut them in half crosswise and remove the seeds. Place in an ovenproof pan and bake at 350°F for 30 minutes. Drop zucchini into boiling water for a few seconds. Drain and season with salt, pepper, and dill. Sauté onions in a little water, the remaining olive oil, and the clove until they are well-cooked and slightly caramelized.

For an elegant presentation, arrange ingredients separately on a serving platter or individual plates with a dollop of yogurt. Or for family style, mix all ingredients together with yogurt.

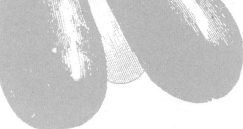

Swiss Chard Stuffed with Barley

4 ounces pearled barley

1–2 bunches Swiss chard (1 large bunch or 2 small)

sea salt to taste

$^1\!/_2$ small onion, cut into small cubes

1 small carrot, cut into small cubes

3 tablespoons olive oil

$^1\!/_4$ small eggplant, cut into small cubes

1 tablespoon parsley

$^1\!/_4$ teaspoon wasabi powder, mixed with
    1 teaspoon water

1 tablespoon lemon juice

❂ *Serves 4–6*

Soak barley in water for 20 minutes, then cook in the soaking water until it starts to split, about 40–50 minutes.

Cut stems of chard and set aside. Drop large leaves in salted boiling water for just a second, to soften. Rinse immediately under cold running water and set aside. Chop stems and small leaves of chard. Simmer onion and carrot in 1 tablespoon oil and a little water.

Soak eggplant cubes for 20 minutes in cold water. Pat dry, season with salt and sauté in 1 tablespoon olive oil. When the eggplant is soft, add other vegetables, barley, and parsley; mix well and adjust seasoning.

Using a small paring knife, remove central vein of the blanched chard leaves, place some of the vegetable mixture in the middle of each leaf, and wrap into a little package. Combine wasabi paste with lemon juice and remaining olive oil and drizzle over lettuce packages just before serving.

✪ ADDITIONAL SUMMER RECIPES ✪

Full information for the books used for these recipes is provided at the end of this section in the Recipe Book Bibliography.

Dr. Haas' Spicy Coleslaw

2 cups green cabbage, grated

1 cup red cabbage, grated

1 cup carrot, grated

$1/2$ cup black olives, diced

$1/2$ small onion, diced, and/or 2 cloves garlic,
 minced and pressed

$1/2$ cup almonds, slivered (optional; for crunch)

2 tablespoons mayonnaise or *Tofunaise* (page 91)

salt to taste

1 tablespoon olive oil

1 teaspoon apple cider vinegar or juice of
 1 medium lemon

$1/4$ teaspoon black pepper

$1/4$ teaspoon red pepper (more for very spicy)

✪ *Serves 4*

Place grated cabbages and carrots in a bowl, and mix in olives, onion, garlic, and almonds (if desired). In a separate bowl, combine mayonnaise, oil, vinegar or lemon juice, and spices, and stir into cabbage mixture. Refrigerate to cool before serving. I served this at my birthday party and it was a big hit!

Fresh Corn and Tomato Soup

from *The New Laurel's Kitchen* by Laurel Robertson,
Carol Flinders, and Brian Ruppenthal

A thick, creamy, coral-colored soup with a truly superb flavor.

$1/2$ onion, chopped

1 stalk celery, chopped

(dash cayenne pepper)

1 whole clove garlic

1 tablespoon oil

5 ears corn (4 cups off the cob)

4 good-sized tomatoes

$1/2$ cup water

$1/2$–1 teaspoon salt

(handful fresh coriander leaves, lightly chopped)

❂ *Serves 4*

Sauté onion, celery, cayenne if desired, and garlic in oil in a heavy 2-quart pan until tender. (This amount of oil will be enough if you keep the heat low and stir frequently.)

Strip corn from cobs with a small, sharp knife. Remove stem end of tomatoes and cut up coarsely.

Add corn and tomatoes, water, and salt to sautéed vegetables. Bring to a boil; then reduce heat to low and simmer, covered, until corn is tender, about $1/2$ hour.

The soup is pretty now, but even better if you take your courage in hand and proceed with the next step: purée it all. Return to pot, thinning with a little more water if you want, and correct the salt. Heat, stirring in coriander leaves just at serving time.

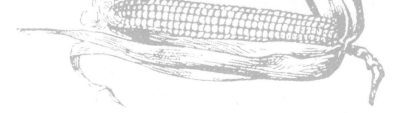

Russian Beet Salad

from *The Enchanted Broccoli Forest (Revised)*
by Mollie Katzen

TIME-SAVER: *Boil the eggs at the same time as the beets; prepare the marinade in the meantime.*

8 healthy (2¹/₂-inch diameter) beets

¹/₄ cup cider vinegar

1 medium clove garlic, minced

2 teaspoons honey

¹/₂ teaspoon salt

¹/₂ cup minced red onion

2 scallions, minced (whites and greens)

1 medium cucumber, peeled, seeded,
   and finely chopped

2 hard-boiled eggs, chopped (Okay to delete yolks)

2 tablespoons minced fresh dill (or 2 teaspoons dried)

1 to 2 cups yogurt or sour cream (or a combination),
   to taste

fresh black pepper, to taste

❂ *Serves 4–5*

Trim the beets of their stems and greens, and place them in a medium-large saucepan. Cover them with water, bring to a boil, and cook until they are tender enough for a fork to slide in easily (about 25 minutes).

Meanwhile, combine the vinegar, garlic, honey, and salt in a medium-large bowl. Stir until well-combined.

Rinse the cooked beets under cold running water as you rub off their skins. Chop them into ¹/₂-inch bits, and while they are still warm, add them to the vinegar mixture. Let stand 30 minutes.

Add all remaining ingredients. Mix well, and chill until very cold.

Israeli Salad

from *The Enchanted Broccoli Forest (Revised)*
by Mollie Katzen

It is best to make this salad in the heart of the Tomato Season. Preparation time is brief, but the salad is best when given an hour or so to marinate before it is served. Chilling is optional—this tastes good at room temperature or cold.
    NOTE: *The ingredients—and their amounts—are flexible.*

6 medium-sized tomatoes, perfectly ripe

2 small (6-inch) cucumbers

5 or 6 radishes, sliced

2 scallions, minced (include greens)

1 large dill or half-sour pickle, minced

1 small bell pepper, minced

1/2 cup green olives, sliced (optional)

1/2 cup minced red onion

1/2 cup (packed) finely minced fresh parsley

3 tablespoons extra virgin olive oil

1 to 2 tablespoons fresh lemon juice
    (optional, to taste)

salt and fresh black pepper, to taste

yogurt to taste (optional)

✪ *Serves 4–6*

Cut the tomatoes in half, and squeeze out and discard the seeds. Cut the tomatoes into 1-inch chunks and place them in a medium-large bowl, along with everything else. Toss gently until well-mingled; taste to adjust seasonings. Serve room temperature or cold.

Tao Salad

from *The Tao of Cooking* by Sally Pasley

3 cups lettuce, torn in bite-
sized pieces

3 sliced raw mushrooms

3 tomato wedges

3 cucumber slices

1/2 cup grated Colby cheese

toasted whole wheat croutons

alfalfa sprouts

Tao dressing

✿ *Serves 1*

Arrange lettuce on a large plate and top with remaining ingredients. Use plenty of croutons, sprouts, and *Tao Dressing* (next recipe).

Tao Dressing

from *The Tao of Cooking* by Sally Pasley

1/3 cup mayonnaise
[*Tofunaise* for lower fat, p. 91]

1/3 cup yogurt

1 1/2 tablespoons cider vinegar

1/2 teaspoon salt

pinch black pepper

1/2 teaspoon finely chopped parsley

1/8 teaspoon basil

1/8 teaspoon dill weed

3–4 spinach leaves

2/3 cup salad oil (cold-pressed
safflower, sunflower, or
soy oil)

✿ *Makes 1 1/3 cup*

Combine all ingredients except salad oil in a blender and purée until smooth. Turn blender on low speed. While motor is still running, slowly pour in oil in a thin stream. When all the oil has been absorbed, turn blender on high speed and blend for a few more seconds to thicken.

Zucchini
with Garlic and Tomatoes

from *The Tao of Cooking* by Sally Pasley

2 tablespoons olive oil

1 teaspoon or more finely chopped garlic

2 tablespoons finely chopped onion

1 tomato, peeled and chopped

1½ pounds zucchini, sliced in ¼-inch thick rounds

2 tablespoons finely chopped parsley

salt and pepper to taste

2 tablespoons bread crumbs

2–3 tablespoons freshly grated Parmesan cheese

✪ *Serves 4*

Heat oil in a skillet. Add garlic and onion and cook 3 minutes. Add chopped tomato and cook, stirring often, for 5 minutes.

Blanch zucchini 3 minutes in boiling, salted water. Drain well.

Add cooked zucchini to skillet with chopped parsley, and season with salt and pepper. When heated through, transfer to a serving dish and sprinkle with bread crumbs and grated cheese. Serve immediately over rice or with a fish dish.

Rice Crust Pizza

from *Eat Well, Be Well Cookbook*
by Metropolitan Life Insurance Company

3 cups cooked brown rice

2 eggs, beaten (or 2 whites and 1 yolk)

1 15 1/2-ounce jar pizza sauce [or homemade
   Tomato Sauce, page 62]

1 small green pepper, sliced into rings

3/4 cup sliced mushrooms (about 3 ounces)

4 ounces shredded part-skim mozzarella cheese
   (about 1 cup)

1/2 teaspoon oregano, crushed

✪ *Serves 6*

Preheat oven to 400°F. Oil a 12-inch pizza pan. In a large bowl, combine rice and eggs. Spread onto pizza pan, making a 1/2-inch rim. Bake about 15 minutes. Reduce oven temperature to 375°F. Spread sauce evenly over crust. Top with pepper rings and mushrooms. Sprinkle with cheese and oregano. Bake about 10–15 minutes until cheese melts.

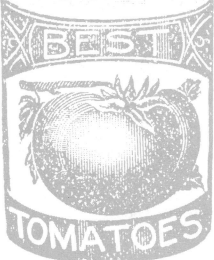

Couscous Casserole

from *Stress, Diet, and Your Heart*
by Dean Ornish, M.D.

2 cups broccoli florets

4 ripe tomatoes, peeled (see Note)

1 teaspoon safflower oil, plus additional for
  baking dish

1 onion, diced

1 clove garlic, minced or put through a press

1 teaspoon grated fresh ginger

$1/2$ pound (2 cakes) tofu, diced

1 teaspoon paprika

2 tablespoons vinegar

1 tablespoon mild-flavored honey

3 cups cooked couscous ($1^1/2$ cups raw)

✿ *Serves 6–8*

Steam the broccoli 5 minutes, drain, and refresh under cold water. Set aside.

Slice two tomatoes and set aside. Purée the rest in a blender or food processor.

Heat the 1 teaspoon oil in a heavy-bottomed skillet and add the onion and garlic. Sauté until the onion begins to soften. Add the ginger, tofu, tomato purée, paprika, vinegar, and honey. Simmer this mixture together over a medium flame, uncovered, for 10–15 minutes.

Preheat the oven to 325°F.

Toss together the tomato-tofu mixture and the couscous. Fill a lightly oiled 2- or 3-quart baking dish with this mixture. Decorate the top with alternating rows of sliced tomatoes and broccoli. Cover with foil or a lid, and heat in oven for 20–30 minutes.

NOTE: To peel tomatoes, drop into boiling water for 20 seconds, drain, and run under cold water.

Pasta with Marinated Vegetables

from *Still Life With Menu* by Mollie Katzen

3 red or yellow bell peppers

12 medium-sized fresh mushrooms, cleaned, stemmed,
and sliced

2 6-ounce jars marinated artichoke hearts (including
all their liquid)

15–20 cherry tomatoes, halved

12–15 large fresh basil leaves, minced (easiest to
use scissors)

3–4 cloves garlic, minced

³/₄ teaspoon salt

6 tablespoons olive oil

2 tablespoons red wine vinegar

12–15 oil-cured olives, pitted and minced

1 pound fettucine or a tubular-shaped pasta
like penne

¹/₂ cup grated Parmesan, Romano, or Asiago cheese

❁ *Serves 4–6*

Preheat oven to 350°F. Place the peppers on a baking sheet and roast for 20–30 minutes, turning every 5–8 minutes or so, until the skin is fairly evenly blistered all over.
Remove from the oven, and immediately place in a plastic or paper bag for about 5
minutes. Remove from the bag. When they are cool enough to handle, peel off the
skin with a sharp paring knife (it should come off easily), and remove stems and
seeds. Slice the peppers into strips, and place them in a large bowl.

Add all remaining ingredients except pasta and cheese, and mix well. Cover and
let marinate a minimum of several hours (24 hours being optimal).

Cook the pasta in plenty of boiling water until al dente. Drain, and combine with
the marinade, adding the cheese as you mix it. Serve immediately.

Banana Yogurt Freeze

from *Fast Vegetarian Feasts*
by Martha Rose Shulman

4 large or 8 small, ripe bananas

1 cup plain, low-fat yogurt

2 teaspoons vanilla, or more, to taste

Freshly grated nutmeg to taste

✪ *Serves 4*

Peel the bananas, cut in chunks, and freeze in plastic bags. They take 24 hours to freeze solid.

Place the yogurt and vanilla in a food processor and add the banana chunks. Using the pulse action of the food processor, process until almost smooth. Then process for several seconds until the mixture is completely smooth. Add nutmeg to taste, adjust the vanilla, and serve. Or hold in the freezer for up to 2 hours (it will become too hard if frozen any longer).

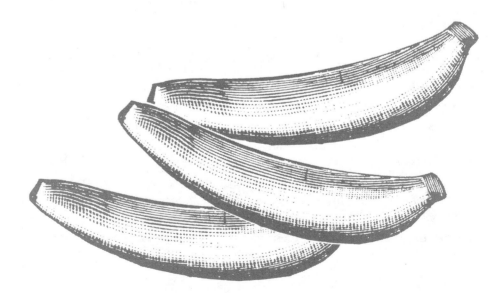

Sunshine Bars

from *The New Laurel's Kitchen* by Laurel Robertson,
Carol Flinders, and Brian Ruppenthal

1 cup orange juice

1 cup dried apricots, loosely packed

$^1/_2$ cup honey

$^1/_2$ cup oil

$1^1/_2$ cups rolled oats

1 cup whole wheat flour

$^1/_2$ cup wheat germ

1 teaspoon cinnamon

$^1/_2$ teaspoon salt

1 cup raisins, partly cut up

$^2/_3$ cup toasted almond meal

❂ *Makes 2 dozen*

Preheat oven to 350°F.

Heat orange juice to a boil. Put dried apricots in pan, bring to a boil again, and turn off heat. Cover pan and let apricots absorb juice until they are tender enough to cut with a sharp knife, but not really soft.

Meanwhile, mix honey and oil. Stir together oats, flour, wheat germ, cinnamon, and salt.

Drain apricots and add the juice to the honey-oil mixture.

Chop apricots coarsely and stir into dry ingredients along with raisins and almond meal. Combine wet and dry ingredients and press mixture into an oiled 9 x 13-inch baking dish. Bake about 30 minutes. Keep an eye on them! Cookies made with honey brown quickly.

Allow to cool completely before cutting.

SUMMER FOODS*

Fruits

Apricot

Avocado

Berries:
  Blackberry
  Blueberry
  Boysenberry
  Loganberry
  Olallieberry
  Raspberry
  Strawberry

Fig

Grapefruit

Lemon

Lime

Melons:
  Cantaloupe
  Casaba
  Crenshaw
  Honeydew
  Musk
  Persian
  Watermelon

Nectarine

Orange

Peach

Pear

Plum

Prickly pear

Tropical fruits:
  Banana
  Breadfruit
  Cherimoya
  Guava
  Mango
  Papaya
  Passionfruit
  Pineapple
  Zapote

Vegetables

Artichoke

Beet

Bell pepper

Cabbage

Celery

Chili pepper

Chive

Corn (fresh)

Cucumber

Eggplant

Green beans

Green peas

Lettuce

Okra

Parsley

Radish

Rhubarb

Spinach

Squash (soft):
  Crookneck
  Scallop
  Zucchini

Sugar peas

Tomato

Watercress

Beans

Green beans

Sprouted beans

Nuts & Seeds

Sprouted

Grains

Sprouted

---

* These are the foods that are naturally available during the summer season in most areas.

For more information regarding seasonal listings and food use, see *The Seasonal Food Guide* poster and booklet, published by Celestial Arts, Berkeley, CA.

CHAPTER 7
AUTUMN

Autumn is the time for a big shift in energy, climate, and diet. It is the official harvest time, and we are all provided with an abundance of nourishing foods. First, farmers harvest the remaining fruits and watery vegetables; then they gather the harder root vegetables and squashes, and whole grains, legumes, seeds, and nuts. Autumn gives us richer and denser foods to support and fuel our bodies and provide us with the additional heat to protect us from the colder, damper climate. Most autumn foods require more heat to prepare. Our diet should shift toward more cooked foods, whole grains, and the richer protein-fat foods as the weather cools and the days shorten. Fewer raw fruits and vegetables and more complex carbohydrates are now the mainstay of the diet, especially from later autumn into early spring.

Autumn is a particularly important time to focus on your health. With more cooked foods, more calories, fats, and proteins, there are often a few added pounds. With this said, a regular exercise program is important for staying healthy in autumn. Focus on indoor activities to maintain physical fitness; for a variety of equipment, join an exercise club. Include daily stretching to maintain or improve flexibility during this more contractive time. Learn to relax and handle the stresses of work, school, and life in general.

The transition into autumn is also a good time for a few days of cleansing with fresh fruits and vegetables, such as apples, grapes, tomatoes, and fresh corn. *The Detoxification Diet* discussed in Chapter 10 offers a smooth transition into improved health. Chew your food well and take time to nourish yourself during this busy season.

❧ AUTUMN MENU PLAN ❧

❧ DAY 1 ❧

Fruit: Apple

Breakfast: Oatmeal with yogurt, raisins, and maple syrup

Lunch: *Fillet of Sole Florentine*
Baked or steamed carrot and beet mélange served over steamed beet tops with a splash of olive oil, lemon juice, and sea salt

Snack: Granola

Dinner: *Lasagna*
Salad greens with vinaigrette

Snack: Baked apple

❧ DAY 2 ❧

Fruit: Grapes

Breakfast: Twice-cooked rice with *Prune and Apricot Compote*

Snack: Pumpkin seeds

Lunch: Baked potato with *Avo-Miso-Tofu Topping*
Grated carrots
Red and green cabbage salad with vinaigrette sprinkled with toasted sunflower seeds or sliced hard-boiled egg

Snack: Soaked prunes

Dinner: Brown rice with adzuki beans
Steamed broccoli and cauliflower with *Walnut-Miso Sauce*

Snack: *Carob-Tofu Mousse*

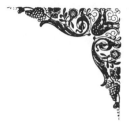

❧ DAY 3 ❧

Fruit: Cantaloupe or other melon

Breakfast: Cornflakes, cooked millet, or
Millet Breakfast Cake with Orange Sauce

Snack: Filberts or pecans

Lunch: *Mushroom Turkey Breast*
Wilted Spinach Salad

Snack: Blackberries

Dinner: *Millet Croquettes*
Brazilian Feijoada (black beans)
Salad greens

Snack: Popcorn

❧ DAY 4 ❧

Fruit: Pear

Breakfast: Cream of wheat or whole wheat toast with peanut-apple butter

Snack: Walnuts

Lunch: *Grilled Swordfish with Pineapple Mustard*
Warm Red Cabbage Salad

Snack: Apple

Dinner: *Pasta alla Boscaiola*
Salad greens with lemon and olive oil

Snack: *Pears in Black Cherry Juice*

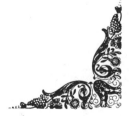

NOTE: Autumn Menu Plan recipes in italics follow in the order listed.

Fillet of Sole Florentine

6 sole fillets

1 tablespoon fresh oregano

sea salt to taste

6 teaspoons lemon juice

6 tablespoons dry white wine (optional)

3 cups fresh spinach, chopped

$1/4$ teaspoon grated nutmeg

lemon wedges

∾ *Serves 6*

Preheat oven to 350°F.

Place fillets in baking dish and sprinkle with oregano, salt, lemon juice, and wine. Bake for 5 minutes. Remove from oven and add spinach and grated nutmeg. Return to oven and bake an additional 3–4 minutes, or until spinach is wilted. Serve with wedge of lemon.

Lasagna

2 tablespoons olive oil

1 cup minced shallots

1 bunch spinach, chopped

1 teaspoon nutmeg

12 lasagna noodle strips, cooked al dente
(slightly undercooked) and drained

6 cups tomato sauce

2 cups leftover cooked beans

1 cup ricotta cheese, or 1 cup tofu mashed together
with 1 tablespoon light miso

sea salt to taste

freshly ground black pepper to taste

Serves 6

Preheat oven to 350°F.

Heat oil in skillet and sauté shallots until transparent. Combine with spinach and nutmeg, and cook 2 minutes.

In a large baking dish, layer lasagna strips, tomato sauce, beans, spinach mixture, and ricotta, until lasagna is used up. Season with salt and pepper. Finish with a layer of tomato sauce and top with ricotta cheese. Cover and bake at 350°F for 20 minutes.

Prune and Apricot Compote

12 cups water

pinch of salt

3 cups prunes, pitted

3 cups dried, unsulfured apricots

1 tablespoon grated lemon rind

❧ *Serves 6*

Bring water and salt to a boil. Add prunes, apricots, and lemon rind; cover and simmer for 1 hour, adding more water if necessary. Serve fruits in their juice.

Avo-Miso-Tofu Topping

1 large, ripe avocado, seeded and peeled

¹/₂ cup tofu, crumbled

1 tablespoon light miso

2 tablespoons lemon juice

1 teaspoon Worcestershire sauce

¹/₂ teaspoon Tabasco sauce

❧ *Makes 2 cups*

Blend all ingredients together until smooth and creamy.

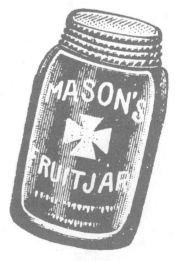

Walnut-Miso Sauce

1 cup roasted (or raw) walnut pieces

1 tablespoon light miso, or to taste

1 tablespoon rice vinegar

½ tablespoon stoneground mustard

4 tablespoons water

½ teaspoon maple syrup or honey

❧ Makes 2 cups

Blend all ingredients together until smooth.

Carob-Tofu Mousse

1 pound firm tofu

2 tablespoons almond butter

3 tablespoons maple syrup

1 tablespoon vanilla extract

¼ cup water

3 tablespoons grain coffee (Peru, Postum, Cafix)

6 tablespoons toasted carob powder

❧ Serves 6

Blend tofu with almond butter, maple syrup, and vanilla until creamy.

Bring water to a boil and dissolve grain coffee and carob powder in it. Mixture should have the consistency of a cream. Add to tofu mixture and blend again until very smooth. Serve in individual parfait glasses.

Millet Breakfast Cake
with Orange Sauce

1 tablespoon corn oil

1 cup dry millet

3 cups apple juice

¼ teaspoon salt

¾ cup shredded coconut

1 tablespoon vanilla

½ cup raisins

∾ *Serves 6*

Preheat oven to 350°F.

Oil a 2-quart casserole. Combine millet, juice, and salt in a saucepan and bring to a boil. Remove from heat and blend coconut with some of the millet and juice. Return to heat and add remaining ingredients. Simmer a few minutes, pour into casserole and bake for 45–60 minutes, or until firm. Allow to cool before cutting, or serve in Pyrex dish.

Serve with *Orange Sauce* (next recipe).

Orange Sauce

2 cups orange juice

½ teaspoon grated orange rind

½ teaspoon grated ginger

pinch of salt

¼ cup maple syrup

1½ tablespoons kudzu dissolved in
   2 tablespoons cold water

∾ *Makes 2 cups*

Bring orange juice, orange rind, ginger, salt, and maple syrup to a boil. Add dissolved kudzu and stir over low flame until thickened.

Mushroom Turkey Breast

3 tablespoons olive oil

herb salt to taste

1 teaspoon thyme

1 teaspoon marjoram

6 turkey breast fillets

1 medium onion, finely chopped

1 celery stalk, finely chopped

3 cups mushrooms, sliced

3 tablespoons dry white wine (optional)

freshly ground pepper

∾ *Serves 6*

Heat oven to 350°F.

Combine olive oil, salt, and herbs. Place turkey breasts in a roasting pan and baste with oil/herb mixture. Bake at 350°F for 10 minutes, basting when necessary. Remove turkey from oven, turn over, and repeat procedure for another 10 minutes or until done, depending on thickness of fillets.

In a skillet, sauté onion and celery over medium heat until onion is limp and transparent. Add mushrooms, stir, and sauté for a few minutes; add wine if desired and cook for 5 minutes longer.

Top each turkey fillet with the mushroom mixture.

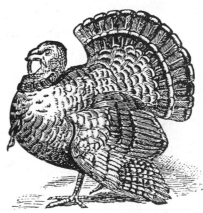

Wilted Spinach Salad

3 bunches spinach (about 12 cups), coarsely chopped

1 red onion, sliced into rings

1 red bell pepper, chopped

6 tablespoons olive oil

2 tablespoons balsamic vinegar

sea salt to taste

1 cup feta cheese, crumbled (optional)

$^1/_2$ cup roasted walnut pieces (optional)

∽ *Serves 6*

Rinse spinach and place in a pot or skillet over medium flame and stir until just limp; it should be bright green. Combine with onion rings and pepper, and toss with oil, vinegar, and salt to taste. Sprinkle feta and walnut pieces on top and serve warm.

Millet Croquettes

3 cups cooked millet

2 tablespoons soy sauce

1 small onion, grated

2 carrots, grated

$^1/_2$ cup parsley, minced

2 egg whites, beaten

∽ *Serves 6*

Combine all ingredients and mash together well. Form into flat 2-inch patties and bake for 5 minutes. Remove from oven and using a spatula, turn patties over, and bake for another 5 minutes or until golden.

Brazilian Feijoada

1–2 tablespoons olive or canola oil

1 large onion, chopped

2 cloves garlic, minced

2 stalks celery, chopped

2 carrots, chopped

4 cups black beans, cooked

1 large tomato, seeded and chopped

1 bay leaf

1 teaspoon ground coriander

1 cup red wine (optional)

1 cup soup stock

tamari to taste

1/4 teaspoon cayenne pepper

∾ *Serves 6*

In a heavy-bottomed pot, heat oil and sauté onion, garlic, celery, and carrots over medium flame, stirring constantly until onion is transparent and limp.

Add beans, tomato, bay leaf, coriander, and wine (if desired). Cook uncovered for a few minutes. Add stock, cover, and simmer for 15 minutes or until liquid is almost absorbed. Remove 1 cup of beans, blend or mash, and return to pot. Season with tamari and cayenne.

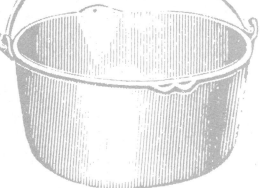

Grilled Swordfish
with Pineapple Mustard

1 tablespoon tamari

1 tablespoon lemon juice

1 tablespoon grated fresh ginger

6 swordfish steaks

1 cup pineapple chunks

1 tablespoon whole grain (stone-ground) mustard

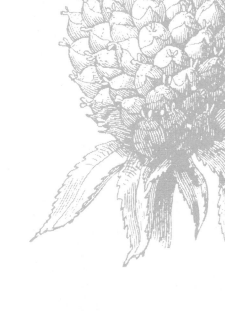

≈ *Serves 6*

Combine tamari and lemon juice in a bowl. Through a cheesecloth or garlic press, squeeze the juice from the grated fresh ginger into the bowl. Dribble mixture over fish steaks and broil for 5 minutes. Turn fish over, dribble sauce over other side, and broil another 5 minutes or more, depending on thickness of steaks.

In a blender or food processor, purée the pineapple with the mustard. When fish is done, remove from the oven and spread a tablespoon of the pineapple mixture on top of each steak.

Warm Red Cabbage Salad

1 head red cabbage

1 small onion, sliced

$1/2$ cup sweet peas, fresh or frozen

5 tablespoons olive oil

3 tablespoons rice vinegar

1 tablespoon ume vinegar or sea salt to taste

$1/2$ cup roasted walnuts (optional)

❧ *Serves 4–6*

Cut cabbage lengthwise into 4 pieces, then slice into $1/4$-inch strips. Steam until soft, about 3–5 minutes.

Sauté onion until limp and transparent and add to cabbage. Add peas, which will cook with the heat of the cabbage.

Combine olive oil, rice vinegar, and ume vinegar or sea salt and toss with cabbage. Sprinkle roasted walnuts on top and serve warm.

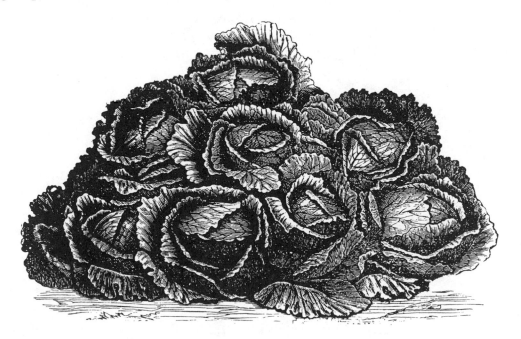

Pasta alla Boscaiola

¹/₈ pound dried cepes or shiitake mushrooms

1 onion, chopped

2 cloves garlic, minced

¹/₂ pound fresh mushrooms

1¹/₂ pounds tomatoes, peeled, seeded, and chopped

sea salt to taste

1¹/₂ pounds whole wheat pasta (spirals or
    other short pasta)

3 tablespoons olive oil

3 tablespoons parsley, chopped

∾ *Serves 6*

Soak dried mushrooms in water for 30 minutes. Drain and chop. (Save soaking water to add to soups or to make risotto.) In a skillet, sauté onion and garlic over medium flame, stirring constantly until onion is transparent. Add fresh mushrooms and cook for 5 minutes. Add soaked mushrooms and tomatoes. Season with salt and simmer, covered, for 20 minutes or until cooking water has evaporated.

Cook pasta in water and salt. Strain, add mushroom sauce, olive oil, and parsley, and mix.

Pears in Black Cherry Juice

6 firm pears

8 cups black cherry juice

1/4 cup fresh ginger, peeled and cut into
   matchsticks (or grate 1 tablespoon ginger and
   press out into cherry juice)

5 tablespoons kudzu diluted in
   6 tablespoons cold water

6 sprigs mint

∽ *Serves 6*

Place pears and ginger in heavy-bottomed pot and pour juice over them. The juice should half-cover them. Cover and simmer until pears are soft but not mushy. Pierce with a toothpick to see if they are done. Remove pears from pot and place on a serving platter or on individual plates. Add dissolved kudzu to simmering juice and stir until thickened. Pour 1 cup of the sauce over each pear and garnish with a mint sprig.

❖ OTHER AUTUMN RECIPES ❖
FROM ELEONORA

Simple Potato and Tomato Casserole

1 pound medium potatoes

1 pound firm ripe tomatoes

2 tablespoons olive oil

sea salt to taste

oregano to taste

grated parmesan cheese (optional)

∾ *Serves 4–6*

Preheat oven to 350°F.

Peel potatoes, slice into ½-inch slices, and steam for 6–7 minutes. Slice tomatoes into ½-inch slices. Oil an ovenproof dish and place a layer of potatoes on the bottom. Season with salt and oregano and place a layer of tomatoes on top of potatoes. Keep layering potatoes and tomatoes, finishing with a layer of tomatoes. Drizzle with a little olive oil and parmesan cheese if desired, add a last pinch of salt and oregano, and bake at 350°F for 20 minutes. Allow casserole to sit for a few minutes before serving.

Chicken and Tomatillos

2 tablespoons olive oil

2 tablespoons vinegar

sea salt to taste

1 teaspoon cilantro, minced

8–10 tomatillos, depending on size, sliced

1½ pounds chicken cut into small pieces

Serves 4–6

Blend together 1 tablespoon oil, vinegar, salt, and cilantro and drizzle over tomatillos. Allow to marinate for 1 hour. Transfer to a pot and cook for a few minutes over medium-low heat. Heat remaining oil in a pan and quickly sauté chicken. Add chicken to tomatillos, and cook covered for 45 minutes. Check seasoning after 15 minutes and adjust if needed.

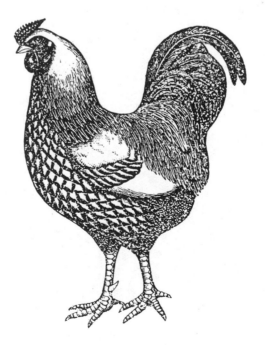

Reduced-Fat
Parsley Mashed Potatoes

1 pound potatoes, peeled

1¼ quarts vegetable stock

sea salt to taste

1 tablespoon parsley, minced

1 tablespoon butter

⌒ *Serves 4–6*

Place potatoes in a heavy-bottomed saucepan and cover with cold vegetable stock. Bring to a boil, cover, and simmer for about half an hour or until cooked through (pierce with toothpick to see if they are done). In a small pan, bring a little water and salt to a boil and blanche parsley for just a moment. Remove from heat, drain, and rinse under cold water. Place a small potato in a blender with the parsley and blend together. Mash remaining potatoes with potato masher, add parsley blend, cook over low heat for 5 minutes and mash to desired consistency, adding more vegetable stock if needed. Finish with butter and season to taste.

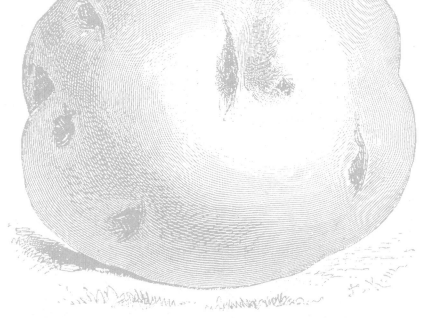

Sea Bass
with Seasonal Pepper Coulis

4 red or yellow peppers

3 tablespoons minced shallots

2 cloves garlic, minced

1 tablespoon fresh thyme

1 tablespoon safflower or canola oil

4 cups court bouillon ($\frac{1}{2}$ stock and $\frac{1}{2}$ white wine)

sea salt to taste

pepper to taste

4–6 pieces sea bass, depending on size

☙ *Serves 4–6*

Cut peppers in half and remove seeds; cut into pieces. Slowly cook shallots, garlic, and thyme in oil until shallots are translucent, about 8 minutes. Place pepper pieces in a heavy-bottomed saucepan with 2 cups court bouillon and simmer for 20 minutes. Purée in blender or food processor with garlic and shallots. Season to taste. Heat remaining court bouillon in a pot with a steamer; season fish and steam until done (time varies according to thickness of fish—check with a toothpick or pointed knife). Serve pepper coulis on individual plates or on a serving platter and place fish on top. Garnish with a sprig of thyme.

◌ ADDITIONAL AUTUMN RECIPES ◌

Full information on books used for these additional autumn recipes are noted in the Recipe Book Bibliography at the end of this section.

Dr. Haas' Split Pea Soup

2 cups green split peas

1 onion, chopped

1 large or 2 medium carrots, sliced

2–3 cloves garlic, minced or pressed

1 tablespoon oil, safflower or peanut (optional)

8 cups water

$1/4$ teaspoon sea salt

black or red pepper, cumin, or curry powder
   to taste (optional)

1 tablespoon miso (optional)

2 tablespoons parsley, chopped

◌ *Serves 6*

Rinse peas. Lightly sauté onion, carrot, and one clove minced garlic in oil in soup pot, add water and peas, then bring to boil. Simmer on low heat for 30 minutes. Add remaining pressed garlic and seasonings. Simmer another 30 minutes or until carrots are soft. If adding miso, dissolve in small amount of water and stir into soup at end. Serve with parsley.

For a more complete meal, add 2 cups of cooked rice to pot at midway, or make croutons from whole grain bread by cubing several slices and baking them at 350°F for 15–20 minutes. Serve with a large green salad.

Kasha Cream
with Sunflower Seeds

from *The Book of Whole Meals*
by Annemarie Colbin

1 cup kasha (buckwheat groats)

4 cups water (or more for thinner consistency)

¹/₂ teaspoon sea salt

¹/₂ cup sunflower seeds

shoyu (natural soy sauce) to taste

✎ *Serves 4*

Grind the kasha in a blender, coffee mill, or handmill. In a 2-quart sauce pan, blend the kasha with 1 cup water until smooth, then add the remaining water and salt. Bring to a simmer, stirring constantly until it thickens. Cover and simmer for 15 minutes, stirring occasionally and adding water as needed. When the kasha has finished cooking, add the sunflower seeds and serve. Allow each person to season individual portions with shoyu to taste.

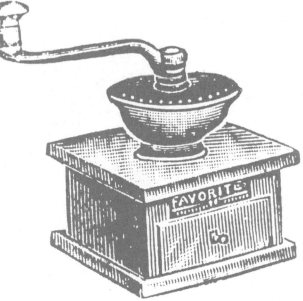

Garlic Soup

from *The Airola Diet and Cookbook*
by Paavo Airola

1½ quarts water

4 potatoes

1 carrot

2 stalks celery

1 onion

2 large bulbs (heads) of garlic

½ teaspoon thyme

dash of oregano

dash of cayenne

sea salt to taste

∾ *Serves 6*

Bring the water to a boil. Cut the potatoes, carrots, celery, and onion into ½-inch pieces, and place in the boiling water. Break the garlic bulbs and peel the individual cloves. Place them in the soup together with the spices. Cook the soup over medium heat for 20–30 minutes. When the soup is ready, it can be served in either of two ways:

- Strain and serve as a clear broth with 1 raw egg dropped into each serving
- Eliminate eggs and purée in the blender and serve as a "cream of garlic" soup

Thai Garlic Soup

from *Still Life With Menu Cookbook (Revised)*
by Mollie Katzen

Don't be scared off by the amount of garlic here! It mellows amazingly as it cooks. The result is a light and gentle first course that can either precede a dramatic entrée or be a soothing, small meal all by itself.

4–5 tablespoons minced garlic

2 tablespoons peanut oil

6 cups light stock or water

4–5 teaspoons soy sauce

1 scant teaspoon salt

3 cups coarsely shredded cabbage

2 medium-sized carrots, cut on the diagonal in 1-inch
   lengths

1 stalk celery, chopped (optional)

a few mushrooms, sliced (optional)

crushed red pepper, to taste (if you go lightly on this
   it lends an intriguing and subtle touch)

❧ *Serves 6*

In a deep saucepan or Dutch oven, sauté the garlic in oil over medium heat until it starts to turn brown. This will take only a few minutes.

Add remaining ingredients and bring to a boil. Lower the heat and simmer, covered, about 10 minutes, or until all the vegetables are tender.

Taste and adjust seasonings. Serve immediately or store for reheating later. Unlike many other soups, this one is not delicate, and reheats readily.

Veggie Burgers

adapted by Dr. Haas from
The Self-Healing Cookbook by Kristina Turner

1 carrot, grated

1 onion, diced

2 teaspoons green onions, chopped fine

1 clove garlic, minced

$^1/_2$ cup chopped parsley or spinach (optional)

2 cups cooked millet, tofu, or cooked soybeans

1–2 tablespoons sesame oil

1 tablespoon tamari

1–2 eggs, beaten

$^1/_2$ cup whole grain bread crumbs

2 tablespoons chopped almonds, peanuts, or
   roasted sesame seeds (avoid for low fat and
   easier digestion)

$^1/_2$ teaspoon thyme

$^1/_2$ teaspoon sea salt

∾ *Serves 4*

Lightly sauté carrots, both onions, garlic, and greens in sesame oil. Transfer to bowl and mix in millet or the mashed soybeans or tofu along with other ingredients. Mix with wooden spoon to a pasty burger consistency, adding water if necessary. Make into patties and sauté in a skillet or, even better, bake in oven on a cookie sheet at 350°F about 40 minutes or until golden brown. Or, form into loaf and bake at 375°F until brown. If desired, melt cheese on burgers and serve with choice of trimmings— buns or toast, sliced tomatoes, lettuce or alfalfa sprouts, catsup, mustard, relish, or *Tofunaise* (see page 91).

Combine with salad, steamed vegetables, corn on the cob, or for a classically American treat, some French fries—but do not fry your potatoes; cut into long strips, like fries, and bake at 350°F until golden brown. Salt lightly and serve with home-made catsup. The kids will love 'em.

Confetti Quinoa

from *The New Laurel's Kitchen*, by Laurel Robertson,
Carol Flinders, and Brian Ruppenthal

Quinoa ("Keenwa"), sacred staple of the ancient Incas, still grows on the high slopes of the Andes—but also, nowadays, on the high slopes of the Colorado Rockies. Quinoa appeals to natural foods enthusiasts for its good nutrition (its balance of essential amino acids is close to ideal) and to gourmets for its unique texture and delicious flavor. Quinoa cooks in just fifteen minutes, and it's so delicate, so light and fluffy, that you can hardly believe it is a whole food. The flavor is appealing, and not quite like anything else, either. It bears some resemblance to couscous, and can be used in much the same way. It shines in dishes where you'd normally use bulgur wheat or millet.

1 cup raw quinoa

2 cups water

¼ teaspoon salt

½ medium onion, finely chopped

¼ each red and green bell pepper, seeded and
  finely chopped

1 teaspoon olive oil

2 tablespoons chopped, toasted almonds or
  ¼ cup sliced water chestnuts

2 tablespoons chopped fresh coriander leaves

◜ *Makes 3 cups*

Rinse quinoa thoroughly in a fine sieve. Bring two cups of water to a boil, then add salt and quinoa and bring to a boil again. Cover, reduce heat to a low simmer, and cook for 15 minutes.

Meanwhile, sauté onion and pepper in olive oil. Combine with grain. Just before serving, stir in almonds or water chestnuts and coriander leaves. Check salt.

Tempeh Cacciatore

from *The New Laurel's Kitchen*, by Laurel Robertson,
Carol Flinders, and Brian Ruppenthal

1 medium onion, slivered

1/2 cup chopped green bell pepper

2 tablespoons olive oil

1 clove garlic, minced

1 cup sliced, fresh mushrooms

2 1/2 cups tomatoes, peeled and chopped

1/3 cup red wine

1 bay leaf

1/2 teaspoon oregano

1 teaspoon basil

8 ounces tempeh, cubed

2 tablespoons shoyu

∾ Serves 4

Sauté onion and pepper in 1 tablespoon olive oil over low heat until onion is translucent; then stir in garlic and mushrooms and cook another 5 minutes or so. Add tomatoes, wine, bay leaf, oregano, and basil and bring to a boil. Reduce heat and simmer for 10 minutes.

Meanwhile, in another small skillet or wok, sauté tempeh in remaining 1 tablespoon oil, stirring frequently, until it browns slightly. Add to sauce along with shoyu, and simmer over low heat to marry the flavors (best if it can simmer at least half an hour). Serve on a bed of whole grain spaghetti or brown rice.

Rich Jalapeño Corn Bread

from *Fast Vegetarian Feasts* by Martha Rose Shulman

For me nothing goes with a bowl of beans better than a thick piece of jalapeño corn bread. This one is almost like cake. You can, of course, omit the jalapeños, and have a delicious regular corn bread. [Also, there is a milk-free corn bread recipe in the Summer section.]

1½ cups yellow cornmeal

½ cup whole wheat flour

¼ cup untoasted wheat germ

½ teaspoon salt

½ teaspoon baking soda

2 teaspoons baking powder

3 large eggs (or 1 yolk and 3 whites for lower fat)

2 cups buttermilk or 1 cup plain low-fat yogurt
   mixed with 1 cup milk

1 tablespoon honey

2–4 jalapeño peppers, seeds removed, chopped

2 tablespoons butter (or corn oil)

ᐁ *Serves 12*

Preheat the oven to 375°F. Place a 9 x 9-inch baking pan or a 9-inch cast-iron skillet in the oven.

Sift together the cornmeal, whole wheat flour, wheat germ, salt, baking soda, and baking powder. In another bowl, beat together the eggs, buttermilk, and honey. Stir in the jalapeños.

Stir the wet ingredients into the dry. Mix together until blended, but do not beat.

Slide out the oven rack holding the hot baking dish or skillet, put in the butter, and return to the oven for a minute. When the butter begins to sizzle, remove the pan from the oven. Using a pastry brush, brush the pan with the butter and pour off any remaining butter into the batter. (Or avoid all butter and just grease the pan with corn oil.) Stir to combine, then pour the batter into the hot baking dish and set in the oven. Bake 30–40 minutes, until the top begins to brown. Cool in the pan, or cut into squares and serve hot.

Szechuan-Style
Sweet and Sour Chinese Cabbage

from *Fast Vegetarian Feasts* by Martha Rose Shulman

This is a provocative dish for those who like spicy food. The miso gives it a satisfying, gutsy flavor.

- 2 tablespoons tamari
- 2 tablespoons vinegar
- 1½ tablespoons mild honey
- 1 tablespoon cornstarch
- 1 tablespoon sesame oil
- 1 tablespoon safflower oil
- ½–1 teaspoon hot red pepper flakes, or dried hot red pepper (seeds removed), minced
- 1 tablespoon miso (optional)
- 2 pounds Chinese cabbage, sliced crosswise into 2-inch pieces
- 2–3 cups hot, cooked grains, such as millet, couscous, or brown rice

ॐ *Serves 4*

Mix together the tamari, vinegar, and honey. Stir in the cornstarch. When it is dissolved, stir in the sesame oil. Set aside.

Heat the safflower (or canola) oil in a wok or large, heavy-bottomed skillet over moderate heat and add the red pepper and optional miso. Stir-fry for a few seconds and add the cabbage. Stir-fry for 2–3 minutes, until the cabbage begins to wilt, then add the tamari mixture. Cook for 1 minute, or until the cabbage is glazed. Serve immediately, with the hot, cooked grains.

Carrot Bread

from *Cosmic Cookery* (out of print)
by Kathryn Hannaford

A good way to use the carrot pulp from making carrot juice.

6 quarts carrot pulp

3 cups honey

1 cup oil

4 cups whole wheat flour

2 cups soy flour

2 tablespoons cinnamon

1 tablespoon nutmeg

4 cups sunflower seeds

4 cups currants or raisins

∾ 4 large or 5 smaller loaves

Preheat oven to 375°F.

Oil a large cookie sheet.

Mix thoroughly carrot pulp, honey, and oil. Sift the dry ingredients together, mix in the sunflower seeds and currants, and add to the carrot pulp mixture. Mix until all flour has been absorbed by carrot pulp. Mold by hand into loaves and bake on oiled cookie sheet at 375°F for about 30–40 minutes.

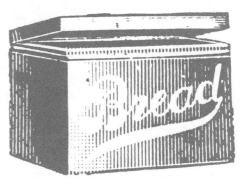

Carrot Hash Browns

from *Fit For Life*
by Harvey and Marilyn Diamond

2 tablespoons butter

1 teaspoon safflower oil

3 medium carrots, peeled and finely grated

3 medium all-purpose potatoes, peeled and finely grated

½ small white onion, finely grated

½ teaspoon sea salt (optional)

∿ *Serves 3*

In large skillet, melt butter and oil. Add carrots, potatoes, and onions. Add seasoning. Sauté until browned on one side. Flip over and sauté on second side until browned. Break apart into small chunks, or serve in wedges cut from the round.

Shrimp Creole

from *Eat Well, Be Well Cookbook* by
Metropolitan Life Insurance Company

4 teaspoons vegetable oil

1/2 cup chopped green pepper

1/2 cup chopped celery

1/2 cup chopped onion

1 garlic clove, minced

1 28-ounce can whole tomatoes, chopped,
including liquid

1/4 teaspoon crushed red pepper

1 bay leaf

1/2 teaspoon thyme, crushed

20 medium shrimp, shelled and deveined (about 10
ounces with shell; 8 ounces cleaned)

1 tablespoon sherry

2 cups cooked rice

Serves 4

In medium saucepan, heat oil over medium heat. Add green pepper, celery, onion,
and garlic and cook about 5 minutes, until tender. Add tomatoes and liquid, red
pepper, bay leaf and thyme; heat to boiling. Reduce heat to low; simmer uncovered
about 30 minutes, stirring often, until reduced slightly. Add shrimp and sherry; cook
about 4 minutes longer until shrimp turns pink. Remove bay leaf and discard. Serve
over rice.

AUTUMN FOODS*

Fruits

Apple

Berries:
  Blackberry
  Cranberry

Date

Fig

Grapes

Jicama

Mandarin
  orange

Melons

Pear

Persimmon

Plum

Pomegranate

Quince

Rosehips

Vegetables

Bell pepper

Broccoli

Burdock root

Cabbage:
  red
  green
  Napa

Carrot

Cauliflower

Chayote

Corn (fresh)

Cucumber

Daikon radish

Eggplant

Garlic (dried)

Gingerroot

Horseradish

Jerusalem
  artichoke

Leeks

Lettuces

Okra

Onions

Parsnips

Potatoes

Pumpkin

Rutabaga

Shallot

Spinach

Squash (hard):
  Acorn
  Banana
  Buttercup
  Butternut
  Hubbard
  Spaghetti

Squash (soft)

Sweet potato

Tomato

Turnip

Yam

Grains (cooked)

Amaranth

Barley

Buckwheat

Corn

Millet

Oats

Quinoa

Rice

Rye

Wheat

Nuts

Almond

Brazil

Cashew

Filbert

Macadamia

Pecan

Pignolia

Pistachio

Walnut

Beans

Adzuki

Black

Blackeye

Carob

Garbanzo

Great Northern

Kidney

Lentil

Lima

Navy

Peanut

Pink

Red

Soy

White

Seeds

Flax

Pumpkin

Sesame

Sunflower

---

* Many foods are available in the autumn harvest. For more information on seasonal eating see *The Seasonal Food Guide* poster and booklet, published by Celestial Arts, Berkeley, CA.

CHAPTER 8

WINTER

Winter is the season for inner nourishing and rest. You may crave richer, more warming foods during this time. Winter meals often require more preparation, and you usually need more fuel to feed your internal furnace for warmth. Perhaps you can spend more time at home, resting, recharging, cooking, and of course, eating. However, watch out for overeating, especially sweets and fatty foods, as decreased activity levels and colder climates can lead to weight gain during this season.

As in autumn, the mainstay of the winter diet are the complex carbohydrates found in whole grains, squashes, and root vegetables such as carrots, beets, potatoes, onions, and garlic. Generally, the winter diet includes more cooked foods, fewer raw foods, salads, and cold drinks. More teas and soups help to keep the body warm. Dairy foods and meats may be consumed more during winter; however, they should never be a very big part of your diet. Fish and high-mineral seaweeds are better rich foods for the winter diet. Poultry may also be consumed more, if you wish.

Winter still requires regular exercise; as in autumn, focus more on indoor activities, with stretching for flexibility. Riding a stationary bike is an excellent aerobic activity. Yoga or tai chi are also wonderful energy enhancers during winter. And, of course, we all need more rest and dream time. This is a season to be close to family and friends, to look at the fire, and stay warm. Be in touch with your emotions and personal healing. Try some special treatments like massage, counseling, or acupuncture to help move those important inner energies which will support your health this winter and throughout your life.

❄ WINTER MENU PLAN ❄

❦ DAY 1 ❦

Fruit: Pear

Breakfast: Sweet potatoes,
Cream of wheat, or
Cracked Wheat with Raisins and Walnuts

Snack: Sunflower seeds

Lunch: *Cream of Broccoli Soup* (optional)
Roasted Turkey with *Mushroom Sauce*
Steamed greens, such as kale or chard

Snack: Mandarin orange

Dinner: *Stir-fried Vegetables with Tempeh or Tofu,*
served over whole wheat pasta

Snack: *Oatmeal Spice Cookies*

❦ DAY 2 ❦

Fruit: Orange

Breakfast: Oatmeal or seven-grain cereal with stewed fruit

Snack: Filberts or pistachios

Lunch: *Curried Chicken Breast*
Coleslaw

Snack: Granola (see page 48 or buy some)

Dinner: *Millet, Squash, and Adzuki Bean Stew*
Steamed kale with olive oil, garlic, and soy sauce

Snack: *Apple-Raisin Compote*

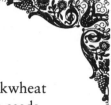

❧ Day 3 ❧

Fruit: Apples

Breakfast: Baked acorn squash with sesame salt, or cream of buckwheat (ground buckwheat, boiled) with raisins and sunflower seeds

Snack: Soaked almonds

Lunch: *Snapper Parmentière*
Arame Carrots, Scallions, and Corn
Steamed greens

Snack: Popcorn

Dinner: *Lentil Soup with Barley and Dulse*
Salad greens and sprouts

Snack: *Pumpkin Pie*

❧ Day 4 ❧

Fruit: Kiwis

Breakfast: Cream of rice with yogurt and honey

Snack: Walnuts

Lunch: *Butternut Bisque*
Poached fish with steamed broccoli and cauliflower or
Norimaki Sushi as a vegetable substitute

Snack: Dates or rice cakes with apple butter

Dinner: *Rice-Lentil Loaf* with *Green Sauce*
Steamed kale or chard with caraway seeds

Snack: Baked apple

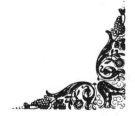

Note: Winter Menu Plan recipes in italics follow in the order listed.

Cracked Wheat with Raisins and Walnuts

2 cups water

1½ cups cracked wheat

1 cup raisins

½ cup walnuts

¼ teaspoon sea salt

½ teaspoon cinnamon

❅ *Serves 4–6*

Combine all ingredients in a pot and bring to a boil. Reduce heat and simmer covered for 40 minutes.

Cream of Broccoli Soup

1 cup water

¼ teaspoon salt

3 cups broccoli, chopped

1 cup low-fat milk

1 cup low-fat yogurt

1 small onion, finely chopped

1 tablespoon light miso, or to taste

❅ *Serves 6*

Bring water and salt to a boil, add broccoli, and cook for 20 minutes. Add milk and yogurt and cook a few more minutes. Purée in blender or food processor with miso.

In a small skillet, sauté onion over medium flame, stirring constantly until golden. Add to soup.

For a nondairy version of the soup, use a very loose rice or oatmeal mixture (1 cup cooked rice blended in 1 cup water or ¾ cup rolled oats cooked in 3 cups water, then blended) instead of the milk and yogurt.

Roasted Turkey

3 tablespoons lemon juice

2 tablespoons tamari

1/8 teaspoon cayenne

1 clove garlic, minced

6 turkey breast fillets

3 tablespoons arrowroot flour

❊ *Serves 4–6*

Combine lemon juice, tamari, cayenne, and garlic in a bowl. Dip turkey fillets in marinade and dust with arrowroot flour on both sides. Place in a baking dish and bake at 350°F until done, about 15–20 minutes on each side (depending on thickness of fillets), basting every five minutes with marinade. Serve topped with *Mushroom Sauce* (next recipe).

Mushroom Sauce

1/2 cup onion, minced

2 tablespoons light oil, such as safflower or canola

6 cups fresh mushrooms, sliced

1/2 teaspoon sea salt or to taste

1/2 cup dry white wine (optional)

1/2 cup chicken or vegetable stock

1 tablespoon kudzu diluted in 3 tablespoons
   cold water

1/2 cup parsley, minced

❊ *Makes 3 cups*

Sauté onion in oil for 5 minutes or until transparent. Add mushrooms and salt and sauté one minute more, stirring well. Lower flame, cover, and simmer for 10–15 minutes. Uncover, add wine, and allow alcohol to evaporate over a high flame for a few minutes. Add stock, lower flame, and add kudzu, stirring until thickened. Adjust seasoning, stir in minced parsley, and serve over *Roasted Turkey* (previous recipe).

Stir-fried Vegetables
with Tempeh or Tofu

8 ounces tofu or 1 pack (6–8 ounces) of tempeh,
   cut into cubes

1 large onion, cut into windowpanes

1 cup fresh (or reconstituted dried) shiitake
   mushrooms

1 cup vegetable stock

2 carrots, sliced on diagonal

1 cup broccoli florets

1/2 cup water chestnuts, sliced

1 cup bean sprouts

1 clove garlic, minced

2 tablespoons grated fresh ginger

tamari or soy sauce to taste

3 tablespoons toasted sesame oil

cayenne to taste

❋ *Serves 6*

If using tempeh, bake or steam for 10 minutes before sautéing. To cut onion into windowpanes, cut in half lengthwise, then cut each half into 3 or 4 sections lengthwise, depending on size of onion. Then slice each section crosswise into 1/4-inch pieces. Remove stems from shiitake mushrooms and reserve to make stock. Slice mushrooms.

In a wok or large skillet, sauté onion in a little water over medium flame until it starts putting out its juice. Add 1/2 cup of stock and bring to a rapid boil over a high flame. Add shiitake mushrooms, cover, and simmer for 5 minutes. Add carrots and sauté for a few minutes, adding stock if necessary; then add tofu or tempeh, broccoli, water chestnuts, bean sprouts, and garlic in that order. Sauté a few more minutes or until broccoli is bright green. Squeeze fresh grated ginger through a cheesecloth and add ginger juice to vegetables. Stir and cook a minute longer. Remove from heat and season with tamari, toasted sesame oil, and cayenne.

Oatmeal Spice Cookies

2 cups whole wheat pastry flour

1 cup rolled oats

pinch of salt

$1/4$ teaspoon allspice

$1/4$ teaspoon nutmeg

$1/4$ teaspoon ginger powder

$1/2$ teaspoon cinnamon

$1/2$ cup water

$1/2$ cup corn oil

$1/2$ cup maple syrup

$1/2$ cup carob chips (optional)

❋ *2 dozen cookies*

Preheat oven to 375°F. Combine flour, oats, salt, and spices in a bowl. Using a whisk, thoroughly mix water, oil and maple syrup. Add liquid ingredients to dry ingredients and mix well to form dough.

Shape pieces of dough into cookies and bake for 10 minutes on each side. For variation, add a half cup of carob or cocoa chips to recipe.

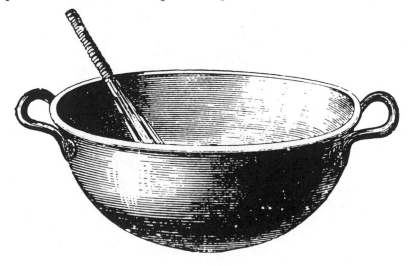

Curried Chicken Breast

1 onion, minced

2 tablespoons safflower oil (optional)

6 chicken breasts

sea salt to taste

1 cup chicken stock

$1/2$ teaspoon cumin powder

$1/2$ teaspoon coriander powder

$1/2$ teaspoon ginger powder

$1/4$ teaspoon asafoetida (optional)

1 tablespoon curry powder

1 cup pineapple, diced

1 tablespoon kudzu, diluted in
    2 tablespoons cold water

❋ *Serves 6*

In heavy skillet, sauté onion in oil until translucent and limp. Add chicken breasts, season with salt, and sauté until golden; turn over and sauté other side until golden. Add $1/2$ cup stock, cover, and simmer until chicken is cooked. Pierce with a fork or paring knife to check for doneness; approximately 5 minutes. Remove chicken breasts and keep warm.

Add cumin, coriander, ginger, asafoetida, and curry to the skillet. Stir and cook until fragrant, about 3–5 minutes, adding the rest of the stock a little at a time.

Purée pineapple and add to sauce. Simmer a few more minutes and add dissolved kudzu to simmering liquid, stirring until thickened. Serve over chicken breasts.

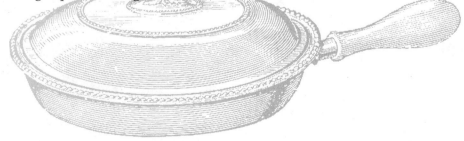

Millet, Squash, and Adzuki Bean Stew

1 cup adzuki beans

1½ cups millet, dry-roasted in skillet

4 cups water

1 piece kombu seaweed

1 small butternut or acorn squash,
  seeded and chopped

tamari to taste

❋ *Serves 6*

Place beans, millet, water, and kombu in a pot and bring to a boil. Reduce heat and simmer, covered, for 30 minutes. Arrange squash chunks on top of the millet and beans. Simmer 30 minutes longer. Season with tamari.

Apple-Raisin Compote

4 apples, cored and chopped

1½ cups apple juice

1 cup raisins

1 cinnamon stick

3 cloves

1 teaspoon grated lemon rind

1 tablespoon kudzu dissolved in
  2 tablespoons cold water

1 teaspoon vanilla extract

❋ *Serves 6*

Bring apples, juice, raisins, cinnamon, cloves, and lemon rind to a boil and simmer until soft, about 15 minutes. Add dissolved kudzu to simmering liquid and stir until thickened; then add vanilla.

Snapper Parmentière

1 medium butternut squash, sliced

1 tablespoon olive oil

sea salt to taste

1 onion, sliced

6 fillets of snapper (or whole fish, 3–4 pounds)

black pepper to taste

4 celery stalks, minced

1 onion, minced

1 clove garlic, minced

1 carrot, minced

1 bay leaf

parsley

1 tablespoon dried thyme

1 tablespoon dried oregano

✳ *Serves 6*

Preheat oven to 350°F.

In a glass baking pan, make a layer of squash slices. Sprinkle with olive oil and salt and top with a layer of onion slices. Rub fish fillets with salt and pepper and place celery, minced onion and garlic, carrots, bay leaf, parsley, and part of the thyme and oregano on top. Roll fillets up and secure with a toothpick. Place them in the baking dish, sprinkle with the rest of the herbs, salt, and ground pepper. Cover and bake for about ½ hour. If using a whole fish, choose a snapper of about 4 pounds, stuff it with the herbs and vegetables, and place it belly down in a baking dish the same size as the fish. Cover and bake for about 1 hour or until fish is done.

Arame, Carrots, Scallions, and Corn

1 package arame seaweed (about 2 ounces)

1 cup carrots, thinly sliced on diagonal

2 tablespoons toasted sesame oil

1 bunch scallions (green onions), thinly sliced
    including green part

1 cup corn kernels

tamari to taste

❄ *Serves 6*

Soak arame in water for about 20 minutes.

In a heavy-bottomed pot, sauté carrots in sesame oil over medium flame for about 5 minutes. Add arame and 1 cup soaking water. Cover and simmer for 20 minutes. Add green onions and corn and season with tamari, then turn off heat and let sit for 5 minutes before serving.

Lentil Soup
with Barley and Dulse

1 tablespoon safflower oil (optional)

1 medium onion, chopped

1 stalk celery, sliced

2 carrots, sliced

1 cup barley

12 cups water

2 bay leaves

2 cups lentils

1 strip kombu seaweed

2 tablespoons dark miso, or to taste

Shredded dulse (optional, or to taste)

❋ *Serves 6*

In a heavy-bottomed soup pot, sauté in oil (or, sauté without oil by using the vegetables' natural juices) onion, celery, and carrots, until onion is limp and transparent. Add barley, water, and bay leaves. Cover and simmer for 20 minutes. Then add lentils and kombu, and simmer for another 30 minutes. Discard kombu and bay leaves. Remove 1 cup of soup and blend with miso. Return to pot. Garnish with shredded dulse.

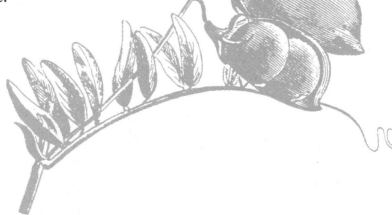

Pumpkin Pie

❧ *Crust:*

²/₃ cup rolled oats

¹/₂ teaspoon salt

¹/₃ cup ground almonds (ground in blender or food processor)

²/₃ cup whole wheat pastry flour

3 tablespoons maple syrup

¹/₂ teaspoon vanilla

2¹/₂ tablespoons water

Mix dry ingredients in food processor. Mix wet ingredients in a bowl. Combine wet and dry ingredients and mix together well. Pat into oiled pie pan.

❧ *Filling:*

2 cups pumpkin, puréed

1¹/₂ cups soymilk

¹/₃ cup maple syrup

1 teaspoon cinnamon

¹/₂ teaspoon ginger

¹/₂ teaspoon salt

¹/₂ teaspoon allspice

¹/₈ teaspoon clove powder

3 tablespoons oat flour, toasted in dry pan

❈ *Makes 1 pie*

Preheat oven to 350°F.

Mix all ingredients together well or blend in food processor. Spoon into pie crust, smooth, and bake for 40 minutes.

Butternut Bisque

1 medium butternut squash, washed thoroughly

7 cups water

$^1/_2$ teaspoon salt

$^1/_4$ teaspoon cumin

$^1/_4$ teaspoon coriander powder

$^1/_4$ teaspoon ginger powder

$^1/_4$ teaspoon garlic powder

6 tablespoons yogurt

$^1/_2$ cup chopped toasted almonds for garnish

❋ *Serves 6*

Cut butternut squash in half, scoop out seeds, and cut into 1-inch cubes. Place in soup pot with water, salt, and spices. Bring to a boil and simmer covered until you can pierce the pieces easily with a fork, about 30 minutes.

Purée soup in blender or food processor, adjust seasoning, and serve with a tablespoon of yogurt in each cup and a sprinkle of chopped toasted almonds.

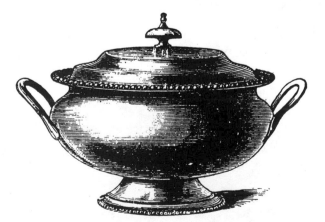

Norimaki Sushi

4 green onions

1 medium carrot, cut into 4 strips

4 sheets of nori seaweed

2 cups pressure-cooked brown rice, or
    1 cup rice overcooked with 3 cups water

2 dill pickles, cut into strips

wasabi (Japanese horseradish) to taste

shoyu (natural soy sauce) to taste

❋ *Serves 4–6*

Bring a little water to a boil in a small pot and quickly blanche green onions and carrot strips.

If you can, find toasted nori in your local health food store or Oriental market. If not, toast each sheet by holding over a flame or baking it in the oven or toaster oven for 2 minutes at 250°F.

Place a nori sheet on a counter or sushi mat and spread about 1/3 cup rice on it, starting closest to you and leaving about 1/4 of the nori at the bottom. Make sure the rice is spread out evenly and reaches the edges of the nori on both sides. Keep a bowl of cold water handy since you will need to moisten your hands frequently to handle the sticky rice.

Lay a green onion, a few carrot strips, and a few pickle strips across the center of the rice layer, making sure the vegetable strips reach the edges. Moisten your hands and lift the sushi mat. Your fingers should be on top of the rice and your thumbs beneath. Roll the mat forward pushing down with your fingers and up with your thumbs. Make sure not to roll the mat into the sushi. When you reach the end of the rice, lightly moisten the nori and seal. Squeeze gently and remove mat. Refrigerate first before slicing, or if serving immediately, carefully slice the roll with a very sharp knife.

Make a paste with the wasabi powder and water and place a dab of it on each roll. Be careful not to use too much since it is very strong. Serve with shoyu for dipping.

Rice-Lentil Loaf
with Green Sauce

1 onion, minced

1 carrot, chopped into small pieces

1 stalk celery, chopped into small pieces

2 tablespoons sesame oil

1 tablespoon rosemary

$^{1}/_{2}$ tablespoon sage

2 cups leftover cooked rice

2 cups cooked lentils or leftover thick lentil soup

2 tablespoons tamari

❋ *Serves 6*

Preheat oven to 350°F.

Sauté onion, carrot, and celery in oil until onion is limp and transparent, then add rosemary and sage and sauté a few minutes longer.

Add rice, lentils, and tamari and mix together well.

Place mixture into an oiled loaf pan and bake covered for 20 minutes. Remove cover and bake another 10 minutes. Let sit for a few minutes before slicing. Serve with *Green Sauce* (next recipe).

Green Sauce

2 cups water

1 tablespoon toasted sesame oil

¼ cup roasted walnut pieces (optional)

4 tablespoons tamari, or to taste

¼ cup finely minced parsley

1 tablespoon kudzu diluted in ¼ cup cold water

❋ *Makes 2 cups*

Bring water and oil to a boil. Add walnut pieces and tamari. Stir in diluted kudzu and simmer until thickened. Add parsley. Serve over *Rice-Lentil Loaf* (previous recipe).

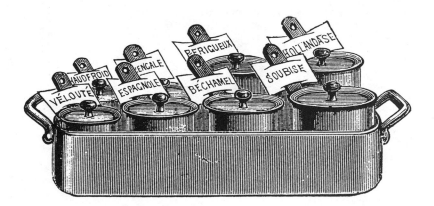

❧ OTHER WINTER RECIPES ❧
FROM ELEONORA

Onion Soup

2 tablespoons olive oil

6 medium onions, finely chopped

1 teaspoon salt

1 tablespoon whole wheat flour

8 cups water

pinch nutmeg

$^1/_2$ pound old bread, cut into cubes

$^1/_4$ pound Swiss or soy cheese, grated

❋ *Serves 4–6*

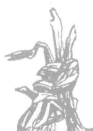

In a heavy-bottomed saucepan, heat oil and add onions. Cover and simmer until onions are very limp, about 15 minutes, stirring occasionally to avoid sticking. Add salt and flour, mix well, and add a small amount of water to dissolve flour and avoid lumps. Add remaining water and nutmeg, cover, and cook 20 minutes. Adjust seasoning. Place bread cubes in ovenproof deep dish, ladle soup over bread, add cheese, and bake for 10 minutes at 350°F.

Leeks and Cauliflower
with Bechamel

9 medium leeks, white part only

1 small head cauliflower, cut into florets

1 tablespoon safflower or canola oil

1 sprig fresh thyme (or 1 teaspoon dried)

1/4 pound whole wheat pastry flour or
    unbleached flour

water to desired consistency

sea salt to taste

1 tablespoon tahini

❋ *Serves 4–6*

Cut leeks in half lengthwise and rinse well under running cold water since they tend to trap a lot of soil. Slice into 1-inch pieces and steam with cauliflower for 10 minutes. Set aside. Heat the oil and thyme in a heavy-bottomed saucepan, add flour slowly, and using a whisk, mix well. Remove from heat and add 1/2 cup warm water, mixing vigorously. When mixture is smooth, place on low flame and slowly incorporate more water until you reach the desired consistency. Season to taste, simmer 10 minutes, and add tahini diluted in warm water. Serve over vegetables.

Macaroni and Tofu Au Gratin

2 tablespoons olive oil

1½ pound onion, diced

6 cloves garlic, minced

¼ teaspoon sea salt

2 cups vegetable stock or 1½ cups water and
   ½ cup shoyu

4 stalks celery including leaves, finely chopped

2 teaspoons dried basil

1 pound tofu, cut into 1-inch cubes

4 tablespoons tahini

½ pound macaroni

2 tablespoons bread crumbs

❄ *Serves 6*

In a heavy-bottomed saucepan, heat oil and sauté onion and garlic over low heat for 10 minutes. Season with salt. Add ½ cup vegetable stock or water and shoyu; cover and simmer for 20 minutes. Add chopped celery, basil, and tofu, and cook 5 more minutes. Dissolve the tahini in ½ cup vegetable stock and add to vegetables. Add remaining vegetable stock. Cook macaroni in plenty of salted water, drain, rinse under cold running water, and add to vegetables. Mix well.

Preheat oven to 400°F. Transfer macaroni and vegetable mixture to an oiled ovenproof dish, sprinkle with bread crumbs, and bake for 10–15 minutes or until top is golden. Serve immediately.

Stuffed Baked Apples

6 large sweet apples, such as Fuji

1 tablespoon raisins

2½ tablespoons tahini

1 teaspoon miso

1 cup apple juice

❄ *Serves 6*

Preheat oven to 350°F.

Core unpeeled apples, leaving bottom part attached. In a blender, combine raisins with tahini and miso. Add a little water if too thick. Stuff apples with raisin mixture and place in an ovenproof dish. Add the apple juice to the bottom of the dish and bake for 30 minutes.

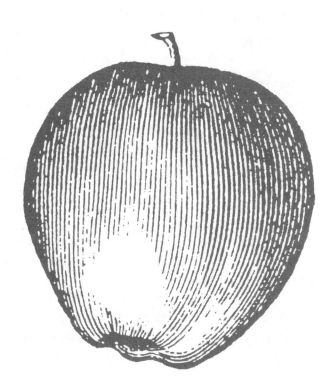

❄ ADDITIONAL WINTER RECIPES ❄

Full information on the books used for these additional winter recipes is provided at the end of this section in the Recipe Book Bibliography.

Russian Soup

from *The Book of Whole Meals*
by Annemarie Colbin

½ cup chickpeas (garbanzos)

½ cup kidney beans

1 cup barley

8 cups water

1 onion

1 carrot

1 turnip

¼ small head cabbage, shredded

2 tablespoons corn or sesame oil

1 teaspoon sea salt

2 tablespoons shoyu (natural soy sauce), or to taste

1 handful parsley, chopped

❄ *Serves 4*

Wash the chickpeas and beans separately, then soak each separately in 2 cups cold water for 8 hours; or bring to a boil, simmer for 2 minutes, and allow to soak in the warm water for 2 hours.

Drain beans; add fresh water to cover. Bring beans and chickpeas to a boil; reduce heat, cover, and simmer for 30 minutes. Then combine the beans and chickpeas with their cooking water in a 4- to 6-quart pot. Add the barley and remaining 4 cups of water; cover and bring to a simmer, cooking for 40 minutes.

Chop the onion, dice the carrot and turnip, and shred the cabbage. Heat the oil in a large skillet over medium heat; add the onion and sauté, then add the rest of the vegetables, stirring well after each addition. Continue to sauté for 10–15 minutes. Now stir the vegetable mixture into the beans and barley; add more water if needed, and simmer for 25 minutes. Season. Garnish the soup with chopped parsley and serve.

NOTE: For cabbage leaves to be tender, this recipe may need to be baked longer. However, the presteaming will usually be enough.

Russian Cabbage Borscht

from *Moosewood Cookbook (Revised)*
by Mollie Katzen

1½ cups thinly sliced potato

1 cup thinly sliced beets

4 cups water

1 to 2 tablespoons butter

1½ cups chopped onion

1 scant teaspoon caraway seeds

1½ teaspoons salt (or more, to taste)

1 stalk celery, chopped

1 medium-sized carrot, sliced

3 to 4 cups shredded cabbage

freshly ground black pepper

1 teaspoon dill (plus extra, for garnish)

1 to 2 tablespoons cider vinegar

1 to 2 tablespoons brown sugar or honey

1 cup tomato purée

❧ *Toppings*:

sour cream or yogurt, extra dill

❄ *Serves 4–6*

Place potatoes, beets, and water in a medium-sized saucepan. Cover, and cook over medium heat until tender (20–30 minutes).

Meanwhile, melt the butter in a kettle or Dutch oven. Add onion, caraway seeds, and salt. Cook over medium heat, stirring occasionally, until the onions are translucent (8–10 minutes).

Add celery, carrots, and cabbage, plus 2 cups of the cooking water from the potatoes and beets. Cover, and cook over medium heat until the vegetables are tender (another 8–10 minutes).

Add the remaining ingredients (including all the potato and beet water), cover, and simmer for at least 15 more minutes. Taste to correct seasonings, and serve hot, topped with sour cream or yogurt and a light dusting of dill.

Hot and Sour Soup

from *Fast Vegetarian Feasts* by Martha Rose Shulman

This soup is a favorite of mine, and one of the easiest and best I know of. It's light and warms you with its slightly piquant, vinegary broth. Even without the traditional pork (or chicken blood, which is often an ingredient in traditional recipes) it's a true Hot and Sour Soup.

6 dried Chinese mushrooms (about 1 ounce)

8 cups water

4 vegetable bouillon cubes

6 green onions, sliced, white part and
    green part separated

2 cakes (1/2 pound) tofu, slivered

2 tablespoons dry sherry or Chinese rice wine

1/4 cup cider vinegar or Chinese rice wine vinegar, or
    more to taste

2 tablespoons tamari, or more to taste

2 tablespoons cornstarch or arrowroot

1/4 cup cold water

2 eggs, beaten (optional)

1/4 cup carrot, cut in 2-inch matchsticks

1/4 cup bok choy or celery, cut in 2-inch matchsticks

1/4–1/2 teaspoon freshly ground black pepper, cayenne,
    or chili pepper to taste

❋ *Serves 6*

Before you begin cutting the vegetables, place the mushrooms in a small bowl. Bring 2 cups of the water to a boil and pour over mushrooms. Cover and let stand 15 minutes. Meanwhile, prepare the other vegetables.

    Place the remaining 6 cups water and the bouillon cubes in a large saucepan. Drain the mushrooms in a strainer over a bowl and add their liquid to the soup pot. Bring to a simmer. Cut the mushrooms in slivers and add them to the stock, along with the white part of the green onions. Simmer 5 minutes and add the tofu. Simmer 5 more minutes and stir in the sherry, vinegar, and tamari. Dissolve the cornstarch or arrow-root in the ¼ cup cold water. Stir into the soup and bring to a gentle boil, stirring.

Drizzle the beaten eggs into the boiling soup, stirring with a fork or chopstick so that the egg forms shreds. When the soup becomes clear and slightly thickened, remove from the heat. Stir in the pepper (be generous—this is the "hot" part of the soup) and adjust vinegar and tamari.

Distribute the carrots, bok choy or celery, and the green onion tops among the bowls and ladle in the soup. Serve at once, passing additional pepper and vinegar so people can adjust hot and sour to taste.

✹ ✹ ✹ ✹

Hot and Sour Dressing

from *Stress, Diet, and Your Heart* by Dean Ornish, M.D.

- 3 tablespoons sesame tahini
- 4 tablespoons cider or white wine vinegar
- 1 teaspoon hot red pepper powder or flaked red pepper
- 2 tablespoons lemon juice
- 1 teaspoon mild-flavored honey
- 1 tablespoon finely minced or grated fresh ginger
- 1–2 cloves garlic, finely minced
- 1 tablespoon finely minced green onions
- 1 tablespoon safflower oil
- 1 tablespoon chopped fresh coriander (cilantro), optional
- ½ cup water
- freshly ground pepper to taste

❋ *Makes 1½ cups*

In a blender or food processor, blend all the ingredients together until smooth. Refrigerate until ready to use. Shake before tossing with the salad.

Kasha with Mushrooms,
Water Chestnuts, and Celery

from *Fast Vegetarian Feasts* by Martha Rose Shulman

This is the innards for the Cabbage Leaves *(next recipe); or, this recipe can be used by itself as a hearty grain dish.*

1¹/₂ cups buckwheat groats (Kasha), washed

1 egg, beaten

3 cups boiling water

1 tablespoon safflower oil

1 small onion, chopped

1 clove garlic, minced or put through a press

8 ounces tofu, diced (optional; will complement the protein)

1 tablespoon tamari (if using tofu)

2 stalks celery, sliced

1 cup mushrooms, sliced

¹/₂ small can water chestnuts, drained

2 tablespoons sherry

salt and freshly ground pepper to taste

❋ *Serves 4*

Mix the buckwheat groats with the egg, and stir together to coat well. Heat a heavy, dry skillet and add the groats. Stir over medium heat until all the egg is absorbed and the groats are beginning to toast. Add the boiling water. When the mixture comes to a boil, reduce the heat, cover, and simmer 20 minutes, or until the liquid is absorbed. Meanwhile, prepare the vegetables.

When the kasha is cooked, heat the oil in a large, heavy-bottomed skillet and sauté the onion with the garlic until the onion is just beginning to get tender. Add the optional tofu and tamari, and sauté 3 minutes. Add the celery, mushrooms, and water chestnuts, and sauté, stirring for a minute, then add the sherry and sauté 3 minutes. Stir in the kasha, and cook another 2–3 minutes. Season to taste with salt and freshly ground pepper. Serve hot.

Cabbage Leaves Stuffed with Kasha, with Creamy Tofu Sauce

from *Fast Vegetarian Feasts* by Martha Rose Shulman

Just in case you're considering freezing this, don't. The cabbage leaves become like cardboard.

✒ *For the Cabbage Leaves*:

2 cups *Kasha with Mushrooms, Water Chestnuts, and Celery* (preceding rccipc)

12 large green cabbage leaves

✒ *For the Tofu Sauce (makes 1 1/2 cups)*:

8 ounces tofu

1 tablespoon miso

1 tablespoon sesame tahini

1/2 cup plain low-fat yogurt

1 tablespoon lemon juice

pinch freshly grated nutmeg

❄ *Serves 4*

Preheat the oven to 350°F. Oil a 2-quart baking dish. Steam the cabbage leaves for about 3 minutes in a large, covered saucepan or wok, until tender and pliable.

Rinse under cold water and drain on paper towels.

In a blender or food processor, blend together the ingredients for the tofu sauce until smooth.

Place 2 heaping tablespoons kasha mixture in the middle of each cabbage leaf. Spread a teaspoon of sauce over the kasha. Fold in the sides of the leaf and roll up, starting at the stem end. Place seam-side down in the baking dish.

Pour 1/2 cup of water in the dish and cover with foil or a lid. Bake for 20 minutes. Top with the remaining sauce and serve.

NOTE: For cabbage leaves to be tender, this dish may need to be baked longer. However, the presteaming step will usually be enough.

Vegetarian Chili

from *Moosewood Cookbook (Revised)*
by Mollie Katzen

2¹/₂ cups dry kidney beans,
   soaked

1 cup tomato juice

1 cup uncooked bulgur wheat

2 tablespoons olive oil

2 cups chopped onion

6 to 8 large cloves garlic, minced

1 medium carrot, diced

1 medium stalk celery, diced

2 teaspoons cumin

2 teaspoons basil

2 teaspoons chili powder
   (more, to taste)

1¹/₂ teaspoons salt (more,
   to taste)

black pepper and cayenne,
   to taste

1 medium bell pepper, chopped

1 14¹/₂-ounce can tomatoes

3 tablespoons tomato paste
   (half a small can)

❧ *Optional toppings:*

finely minced parsley,
   grated cheese

❋ *Serves 6–8*

Place the soaked beans in a Dutch oven or kettle, cover with water, and bring to a boil. Partially cover, turn heat down to a simmer, and cook until tender (about 1¹/₄ hours). Watch the water level during cooking, adding more if necessary. Drain off any excess water when the beans are done.

Heat the tomato juice to boiling. Add it to the bulgur in a small bowl, cover, and let stand 15 minutes. Add this to the cooked beans.

Heat the olive oil in a medium-sized skillet. Add onion, half the garlic, carrot, celery, and seasonings. Sauté over medium heat about 5 minutes, add bell pepper, and sauté until all the vegetables are tender.

Add the sautéd vegetables, tomatoes (au jus), and tomato paste to the beans. Simmer over lowest possible heat, stirring occasionally, for 20–30 minutes or longer. After about 15 minutes, add remaining garlic. Taste to adjust seasonings, and serve hot, topped with parsley and/or cheese.

Spicy Nut Sauce

from *Dr. Braly's Food Allergy and Nutrition Revolution*
by James Braly, M.D.

- 2 tablespoons chopped green pepper
- 1 small onion, minced
- 1 tablespoon oil
- 1 cup chopped tomato
- $1/4$ teaspoon salt
- $1/2$ teaspoon chopped jalapeño pepper or
  $1/4$ teaspoon cayenne pepper
- $1/3$ cup nut meal (walnuts, pecans, or
  sunflower seeds, ground)
- $1/4$ cup water

❋ *Makes 1 cup*

Sauté green pepper and onion in oil until tender. Add tomato and cook for 5 minutes or until soft. Stir in salt, pepper, and nut meal. Gradually add water, stirring to make a creamy sauce. Heat through and adjust spices to taste. May serve over grain and/or vegetable dish.

Basmati Rice 'n' Eggs

by Bethany ArgIsle

Basmati is known in the East as the "rice of kings." It is light with a flowery fragrance.

3 cups basmati rice

5 cups water

6 eggs

6 green onions, chopped fine

1 small bunch cilantro, chopped fine

3 ripe tomatoes

1/4 cup olive oil

3 tablespoons low salt soy sauce or mineral bouillon

1/4 teaspoon cayenne pepper

2 tablespoons toasted sesame oil

❋ *Serves 4–6*

Rinse rice thoroughly until water is clear. Add fresh water two finger breadths above rice and boil rapidly over moderate heat. Do not burn.

Soft-boil eggs 3–4 minutes; then, run under cold water and peel. Wash and chop separately the green onions, cilantro, and tomatoes; place in individual bowls for personal serving garnish.

Add rice, eggs, oil and all seasonings to large bowl and mix lightly. Taste and balance seasonings as desired. Add garnish according to individual taste.

Leftovers are a lot of fun and can be planned the day before by making more of this dish than needed. Get out your wok or skillet and heat it over a hot flame. Then add first 1/2 cup of purified water or 1/4 cup of olive oil or rice bran oil. Immediately add rice and eggs with any lightly steamed vegetable such as green or red bell or chili peppers—or you can prebroil fresh, organic turkey sausage or soy sausage, chop, and add to dish. Add green onions a minute before dish is done. Cilantro and tomatoes can be used for garnish.

Soya Carob Nut Brownies

from *Cosmic Cookery* (out of print)
by Kathryn Hannaford

2 cups oil

2 cups honey

4 cups water

1 cup coconut

4 cups presifted whole wheat
   pastry flour

2 cups carob powder

1 cup soymilk powder

2 tablespoons baking powder

1 tablespoon sea salt

2 cups walnut pieces

❋ *Makes 30–35 brownies*

Preheat oven to 350°F.
   Oil 1-inch deep cookie sheet lined with waxed paper (9½ x 15 inches).
   Combine the first four ingredients in a large bowl, mixing well. In another bowl, mix together the next five ingredients. Sift the dry ingredients gradually into the liquid ingredients, beating well after each addition. Beat until the batter is smooth, and then fold in the chopped nuts. Spoon the mixture into the oiled cookie sheet, filling it half full (½ inch). Bake at 350°F until a toothpick inserted into the center of each pan comes out clean. Remove to cooling racks before frosting with *Carob Icing* (optional; see recipe below).

Carob Icing

1 cup water

½ cup oil

1 cup honey

1 cup carob powder

1½ cups skim milk powder

½ cup soymilk powder

❋ *Makes 6 cups*

Mix the first three ingredients in a bowl. Sift the last three ingredients into the liquid, one at a time, beating well after each addition. The icing should be thick enough to harden on the cake. It should not be sticky, nor too hard. Add more skim milk powder if necessary.

Tofu Banana Cream Pie

from *Stress, Diet, and Your Heart* by Dean Ornish, M.D.

People often can't believe that they're eating tofu when they eat this low-fat dessert. It's creamy and rich, much like a cheesecake.

1 cup granola

2 teaspoons ground cinnamon

safflower oil for pie pan

1 pound tofu

1 cup nonfat yogurt

1/4 cup apple juice

3 tablespoons mild-flavored honey

2 teaspoons vanilla extract
    (more to taste)

3 large ripe bananas

1/2 teaspoon nutmeg

juice of 1 1/2 lemons
    (more to taste)

3 tablespoons whole wheat flour

1/2 cup fresh strawberries

❊ *Serves 8*

Preheat the oven to 350°F.

Mix together the granola and 1 teaspoon cinnamon.

Brush a 9- or 10-inch pie pan or an 8-inch springform pan lightly with safflower oil and sprinkle the granola evenly over the bottom.

Blend together the tofu, yogurt, apple juice, honey, vanilla, 2 bananas, nutmeg, 1 teaspoon cinnamon, the juice of 1 lemon, and the whole wheat flour in a blender or food processor until completely smooth. Make sure there are no little chunks of tofu left unblended.

Pour into the prepared baking dish and bake in the preheated oven for 50 minutes, until the top is just beginning to brown. Remove from the oven and cool, then chill several hours.

Before serving, slice the remaining banana and toss with remaining lemon juice. Cut the strawberries in half, and decorate the top of the pie with the banana slices and strawberries.

WINTER FOODS*

Fruits

Apples:
  Granny Smith
  Pippin
  Red Delicious

Cranberry

Dates

Dried fruits:
  Apple
  Apricot
  Coconut
  Mango
  Papaya
  Pear
  Peach
  Pineapple
  Prune
  Raisin

Grapes

Jicama

Kiwifruit

Kumquat

Mandarin
  orange

Navel orange

Pear:
  Anjou

Persimmon

Pomegranate

Tangelo

Tangerine

Vegetables

Bok Choy

Broccoli

Brussels
  sprouts

Burdock root

Cabbages

Carrots

Cauliflower

Chard

Daikon radish

Garlic

Ginger

Jerusalem
  artichoke

Kale

Leeks

Onions

Parsnip

Potatoes

Rutabaga

Seaweeds:
  Agar
  Arame
  Dulse
  Hijiki

Kelp
  Kombu
  Nori
  Wakame

Spinach (New
  Zealand)

Sprouts

Squash (hard):
  Acorn
  Butternut
  Delicata
  Hubbard
  Spaghetti

Sugar pumpkin

Sweet potato

Turnip

Yam

Nuts & Seeds

same as
  Autumn

Sprouts

Seeds

Grains

Beans

* These are the foods that are naturally available to many areas during the winter. For the colder and snowy climates, most winter foods must have been dried and stored to provide our nourishment. *The Seasonal Food Guide* poster and booklet, also by Dr. Haas and published by Celestial Arts, gives further information on the seasonal diets.

PART III

SPECIAL DIETS,
DETOXIFICATION,
AND OTHER
HEALTH
GUIDELINES

"One cannot think well, love well, sleep well, if one has not dined well."

VIRGINIA WOLF

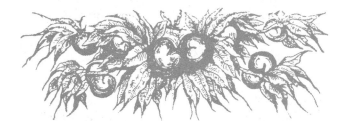

Over the centuries, throughout all cultures, diet has been a very important aspect of health and healing. In this chapter we include a short discussion of four different nutritious eating approaches that have become popular in America over the last quarter century and particularly, over the last decade. We are lucky in this country than we can experiment with different diet choices. Let this chapter be an introduction or "sampling" of healthful diets, one of which may be ideal for you.

- The *Fat-Free Diet* has been popularized by Dr. Dean Ornish and Dr. John McDougall for the prevention and treatment of cardiovascular disease. Fortunately, with more information on the role fats play in causing many of our modern-day diseases, the consciousness of the general public is changing, and the food industry is starting to reflect those changes. Most of the recipes in this book are low in fat, and in this section Eleonora has created a fat-free menu that we think you will find surprisingly tasty.

- The *Natural Hygiene/Raw Foods Diet* is mainly a detoxification program, and adds another dimension to healthy eating. It uses fresh, raw, and natural foods as the mainstay of the diet, avoiding any cooking so as to leave the nutrients, enzymes, and vitality of food intact. This, its advocates claim, leads to health and vitality in the body and mind.

- The *Macrobiotic Diet,* on the other hand, emphasizes a diet of *cooked* whole grains, beans, and vegetables as the bulk of a healthy diet, with the addition of some white fish. Although strict macrobiotics is not for everyone, it has afficionados all over the world and is often helpful in the treatment of chronic disease. A more moderate version of this diet has recently become popular as a transition from the unhealthy Western eating program.

• The *Ayurveda Diet* is part of the ancient healing system of Ayurveda, which is based on a subtle balancing of the different mind/body types *(doshas)*. The diet uses a natural, wholesome, and primarily vegetarian approach to eating. Ayurveda has become more utilized recently in America with the popularity of Dr. Deepak Chopra, a physician and author who teaches this ancient Indian healing system.

For a more in-depth look at any of these diets, consult your local bookstore or health food store. *Staying Healthy with Nutrition* further discusses some of these diets and others that you might be enticed to try. The next chapter in this book, Detoxification and Rejuvenation, offers you a healing and healthful transition from your current diet into one of these other eating programs. Here's to adventures in food!

CHAPTER 9

SPECIAL DIETS

FAT-FREE DIET

There is clearly a relationship between fats in the diet, especially animal fats and hydrogenated oils, and chronic degenerative diseases. High-fat diets are strongly implicated in atherosclerosis and consequent cardiovascular problems, including heart disease and heart attacks—the number one killers in America. Dietary fats are also linked to a variety of cancers, most commonly breast and colon cancers.

Therefore, many people who exhibit these diseases or who wish to prevent them are beginning to eat a very low-fat and high-fiber diet. For this reason, fat-free foods and fat-free recipes and menus are becoming more popular.

Although it is unhealthy to completely avoid all fats and oils due to our need for essential fatty acids, these essential fatty acids need compose only a very small percent of total calories in the diet, and our requirements can easily be fulfilled in a low-fat diet.

The following pages offer you a special selection of fat-free recipes and a sample fat-free menu. As long as you obtain the equivalent of about two teaspoons of good-quality vegetable oils daily, you will fulfill your need for the right oils. Good sources are: fresh raw almonds, walnuts, sunflower seeds, pumpkin seeds, or cold-pressed olive, flax, or canola oil.

Ultimately, you can do a great job at reducing and preventing cardiovascular disease and creating high-level health if you eat a wholesome, balanced diet, engage in regular exercise, and get a handle on the stress in your life. Fat-free eating is one of the most successful ways to maintain a healthy heart.

211

❧ Fat-Free Menu ❧

Crostini with White Bean and Pesto Purée
Small Dinner Salad with Tomato Vinaigrette
Couscous Flan with Parsley-Mint Sauce
Steamed Vegetables with Creamy Garlic Sauce
Bread Pudding

White Bean and Pesto Purée

$^3/_4$ cup white beans, soaked overnight

$^1/_2$ medium onion, coarsely chopped

3 cloves garlic, minced

1 sprig parsley

1 bay leaf

4 cups water

1 cup fresh basil

juice of 1 lemon

sea salt to taste

cayenne to taste

❧ *Makes 2$^1/_2$ cups*

Simmer beans, onion, 2 cloves garlic, parsley, and bay leaf in 3 cups water for 1 hour. Drain and discard bay leaf. Blend with basil, lemon juice, additional clove of garlic and draining water to desired consistency. Season to taste with sea salt and cayenne. Serve over toasted French bread.

Tomato Vinaigrette

juice of ¹/₂ lemon
1 tablespoon balsamic vinegar
1 small clove garlic, minced
¹/₂ teaspoon Dijon mustard
¹/₄ teaspoon dried thyme
¹/₄ teaspoon dried marjoram
1 large tomato, peeled and seeded
sea salt to taste

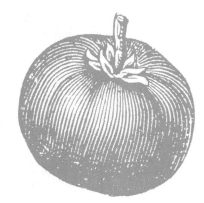

❧ *Makes 1 cup*

Blend all ingredients together and serve over seasonal mixed greens.

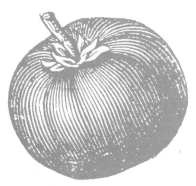

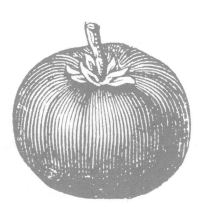

Couscous Flan

3 cups carrot juice

2 cups whole wheat couscous

1/2 teaspoon sea salt

parsley for garnish

❧ *Serves 4–6*

Place carrot juice and couscous into a pot with salt. Bring to a boil, cover, and simmer for 15 minutes. Press cooked couscous into a bowl and unmold onto a serving platter. Decorate with parsley.

Parsley-Mint Sauce

1 onion, finely chopped

1 cup split peas

1 bay leaf

5 cups water

1/4 cup minced parsley

1 tablespoon minced chives

1 tablespoon minced mint

sea salt to taste

❧ *Serves 4–6*

Steam onion in a tablespoon of water until limp; add split peas, bay leaf, and 5 cups water. Simmer for 45 minutes. Add parsley, chives, and mint and simmer 2 more minutes, adding more water if consistency is too thick. Salt to taste and blend in a food processor or blender. This sauce is also very good with pasta, polenta, or rice.

Creamy Garlic Sauce

15 cloves garlic, peeled and left whole

1/8 teaspoon dried sage

1/8 teaspoon dried thyme

1 1/2 cups water

2 tablespoons dry white wine

juice of 1/2 lemon

sea salt to taste

2 tablespoons minced parsley

cayenne to taste

Makes 1 cup

Simmer garlic, sage, and thyme in water and wine for 30–40 minutes. Purée in blender until soft. Add lemon juice and salt. Stir in parsley and cayenne and heat before serving. Excellent over steamed vegetables, baked potatoes, or grains.

Bread Pudding

3/4 pound old bread

4 cups apple juice

1/2 cup raisins

1/2 teaspoon cinnamon

2 apples

Serves 6

Cut bread into cubes and set aside in a saucepan. Bring apple juice, raisins, and cinnamon to a boil and pour over bread cubes. Cover and let sit a minimum of 2 hours, or overnight.

Preheat oven to 450°F. Peel, core, and grate apples, and add to bread. Spray or oil a springform pan and transfer bread-apple mixture into it. Cover with foil and bake for 35 minutes. Remove foil and bake 25 minutes longer. Allow to cool in pan, unmold, and serve. This pudding is even better if prepared a day ahead.

NATURAL HYGIENE/ RAW FOODS DIET

Natural Hygiene is an ancient system of healing, utilizing a raw-foods diet supported by cleansing the colon and occasional fasting. It traces its origins back to the Essenes, an ancient Jewish tribe of scholars, as well as to ancient Greece, and has had followers for many centuries throughout the world.

The dietary philosophy of Natural Hygiene states that one should consume foods as close to their natural state as possible; that is, primarily raw, and if cooked, never at a temperature higher than 100°F. Adherents avoid all animal products, and favor foods that do not involve killing. Fruits are primarily eaten. Vegetables and herbs are considered medicinal as they help to attain or maintain balance. Nuts and seeds also play an important role, mostly in their sprouted form. Fermented juices are considered very beneficial because of their high enzyme content.

The principles of food combining have their origin in the Natural Hygiene Diet. According to these principles, starches and proteins should not be eaten at the same time, since starches need an alkaline pH environment to be well-digested and proteins require a more acid pH. Fruits should be eaten only with other fruits since they transit through the body more quickly than other foods, and if they are detained in the stomach due to the presence of slower-to-digest foods, their fruit sugar will ferment and cause gas and indigestion. (See also pp. 14–15)

Pure air, pure water, sunshine, and daily exercise are also very important aspects of life for a natural hygienist, as are relaxing before and during meals, eating slowly, and chewing well—all of which are crucial to good digestion and assimilation. A peaceful, loving disposition towards all life forms and a positive mental attitude are some of the higher ideals of Natural Hygiene philosophy.

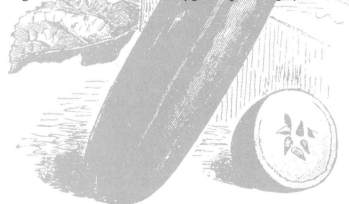

❧ Natural Hygiene Menu ❧

Sweet Corn Gazpacho
Raw Hummus
Sauerkraut
Raw Apple Pie

Sweet Corn Gazpacho

3 cups corn, cut fresh off the cob

3 cups tomatoes, peeled, seeded, and chopped

2 tablespoons parsley, minced

$^1/_2$ cup celery hearts chopped, including tops

1 teaspoon vegetable seasoning
   (see *Seasoning Mix*, p. 44)

1 cup water

1 lemon, sliced

❧ *Serves 4–6*

If using a food processor, briefly process all ingredients, except lemon, using the pulse action. If using a blender, blend for just a few minutes. There should be chunks in this soup. Serve cold with a lemon slice in each dish.

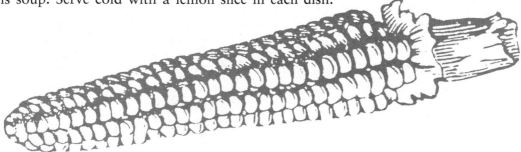

Raw Hummus

3 cups sprouted chickpeas
   (garbanzo beans)

1 clove garlic

2 tablespoons lemon juice

3 tablespoons olive oil

1 teaspoon sea salt

1 tablespoon paprika

◆ Serves 4–6

Blend all ingredients together in blender or food processor, and serve with cucumber slices or Essene bread (sprouted, uncooked grain bread).

Sauerkraut

1¹/₂ large heads red or white cabbage

2 tablespoons kelp powder

2 teaspoons garlic (optional)

2 teaspoons ground dill seed

◆ Makes ¹/₂ gallon

Remove outer leaves of cabbage heads and set aside. Grate cabbage and mix with seasonings. Place in a glass or porcelain container. Avoid plastic or metal. Cover with outer cabbage leaves and place a plate and a weight on top of closed container. Leave at room temperature for five days. Remove foam and leaves and mix so juice is evenly distributed. Store covered in the refrigerator; it will keep for weeks.

Raw Apple Pie*

● *Crust:*

1 cup almonds

$^1/_2$ cup pecans

$^1/_3$ cup chopped pitted dates

3 tablespoons water

● *Filling:*

4 apples, grated with peel

2 bananas, mashed

$^1/_4$ cup lemon juice

1 cup dates, pitted and mashed

$^1/_4$ cup grated coconut

● *Makes 1 pie*

In water, soak almonds and pecans overnight in separate bowls. Drain and rinse.
Preheat oven to 250°F.

In a food processor, grind almonds and pecans separately to a moist meal. Combine in a bowl. Blend dates with water in the food processor and stir into nut mixture until well-mixed and dough-like in consistency. Shape nut mixture into a ball and place on a sheet of waxed paper. Top with another sheet of waxed paper, and with a rolling pin, roll out into a circle 11 inches in diameter.

Remove top sheet of paper and press pie crust gently into an oiled 9-inch pie plate. Bake for 30 minutes, remove from oven, and allow to cool. Combine grated apples, lemon juice, mashed bananas, dates, and coconut; spoon into crust.

---

*We have chosen to add this fruit dessert to the menu, but according to the Natural Hygiene principles, this dish would be eaten two to three hours after dinner, or as a morning fruit meal.

MACROBIOTIC DIET

The Macrobiotic Diet originated in the Zen monasteries of China and was grounded in the ancient principles of yin and yang. Based on whole grains, this diet was thought to be an earthy, grounded eating plan conducive to the practice of meditation. Macrobiotics was also incorporated in Japan and then was brought to America in this century by George Ohsawa. Through the teachings of Michio Kushi and Aveline Kushi, it has gained some popularity over the last twenty years as a healing program to balance the excesses of the Western diet. It has also been used as a protection and possible treatment for cancer. This, and its overall strict nutritional guidelines, have made the macrobiotic approach controversial in the medical community.

A macrobiotic diet consists almost exclusively of cooked foods. Raw foods are thought to be too difficult to digest and too cooling for the body. A minimum of fruit is consumed, and most of it cooked, as in baked apples. Dairy foods and eggs are avoided; the only animal products recommended are whitefish, such as halibut, trout and sole, and these are kept to less than five percent of the diet.

Macrobiotic meals include between fifty and sixty percent whole cereal grains, such as brown rice, whole oats, millet, barley, corn, buckwheat, wheat berries, and rye. Flour products and baked goods are avoided; pasta and breads are eaten only occasionally. Vegetables make up twenty to twenty-five percent of the diet; members of the nightshade family, namely potatoes, peppers, tomatoes, and eggplant, as well as avocado, spinach, yams, and sweet potatoes are all avoided. Beans and sea vegetables are suggested to complement the meals, making up five to ten percent of the diet. The primary beans eaten are adzukis, lentils, and garbanzos, along with fermented soybean products such as tofu, tempeh, and miso. Most other beans can be eaten occasionally in this diet. Some nuts and seeds and vegetable oils may be used. Soups and salads can also be consumed, constituting about five percent of the diet. Other exotic foods like umeboshi plums (and other pickled foods such as daikon radish and ginger, usually eaten at the end of the meal to aid digestion), tamari soy sauce, sesame salt (gomasio), and bancha twig tea are also included.

Overall, macrobiotics can be a fairly balanced eating approach, although I believe it needs more individual and climatic variations. Also, I believe that most of us need more fresh, uncooked fruits and vegetables, especially in the warmer climates. (See previous Natural Hygiene discussion.)

❧ *Macrobiotic cooking methods:*

According to the macrobiotic philosophy, the values and perspective of the cook are transmitted to the people who eat the food, including the way the food is handled and prepared, the sense of composition, and the overall balance of the meal. Depending on the results one wishes to achieve, there are a number of different ways a simple dish such as rice can be prepared. I will try to summarize just a few of the most important rules of macrobiotic cooking.

- Every time you approach the stove, remember that the simplest cooking is usually the best.

- Food should be treated with respect, therefore not ever wasted or handled carelessly.

- It is preferable to use a whole vegetable. Cut vegetables in a mindful way, paying attention to shape and size.

- Use a pressure-cooker for grains and beans: it makes beans more digestible by breaking down the tough cellulose wall that is responsible for creating flatulence in some people, and it also brings out the natural and soothing sweetness of the grains.

- If you are overweight, bloated, premenstrual, or feeling scattered, use a cooking method that removes water from the food, such as grilling, broiling, baking, or sautéing.

- If you feel tight, rigid, self-righteous, or anxiety-ridden, use a cooking method that adds water to the food, such as steaming, boiling, or blanching.

- Choose a variety of foods for your meal. Ideally, you should have a grain and bean combination or a protein food, a vegetable that grows upward out of the ground, and a vegetable that grows downward into the ground. Also, try to have five different colors in your meal.

- Do not use the same cooking method for the whole meal.

❧ MACROBIOTIC MENU ❧

Mushroom Miso Soup
Brown Rice and Adzuki Beans with Arame
Bok Choy in Ginger Sauce
Apple Mousse

Mushroom Miso Soup

3 dried shiitake mushrooms

8 cups water

1 strip kombu seaweed

1 cake tofu, cut into small cubes

2 tablespoons dark miso (barley or brown rice)

2 scallions, thinly sliced

2 sheets sushi nori seaweed, shredded

❧ *Serves 4–6*

Soak mushrooms in 1 cup water for 10–15 minutes. Bring remaining water and kombu to a boil, lower heat, and simmer. Remove mushrooms from soaking water and add soaking water to simmering kombu.

Remove stems from mushrooms and discard. Thinly slice the caps. Add sliced mushroom caps to soup and simmer 10 minutes longer.

Add tofu and simmer 5 minutes. Remove kombu, dissolve miso in a cup of soup, and return to soup pot. Remove from heat and add scallions and shredded seaweed.

Brown Rice and Azduki Beans with Arame

1 cup arame seaweed

2 cups short grain brown rice

2 cups adzuki beans

4 scallions, thinly sliced on the diagonal

tamari to taste

Serves 4–6

Soak arame in water for 20 minutes.

Place rice and beans in a heavy-bottomed saucepan with four times the amount of cold water and a pinch of sea salt. Bring to a boil, cover, and simmer for 50 minutes to one hour.

Drain arame and add to rice with some of the soaking water if necessary. Simmer 10 more minutes. Add sliced scallions and season with tamari.

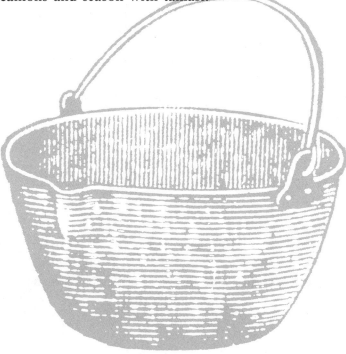

Bok Choy in Ginger Sauce

3 bok choy or 6 baby bok choy

1 tablespoon toasted sesame oil

2 cloves garlic, minced

1 tablespoon grated ginger

1 teaspoon kudzu

2 tablespoons tamari, or to taste

❧ *Serves 4–6*

Slice bok choy into 1-inch strips. Separate white part from leaves. Heat oil in a skillet and sauté garlic with white part of bok choy for a few minutes. Add leaves and sauté a few more minutes.

Wrap grated ginger in a cheesecloth and press juice into the vegetables. Dilute kudzu in 2 tablespoons cold water and add to vegetables, stirring to coat. Season to taste with tamari and remove from heat.

Apple Mousse

7 cups apple juice

7 teaspoons agar-agar flakes

1 tablespoon tahini

cinnamon to garnish

❧ *Serves 4–6*

Bring apple juice and agar-agar to a boil, and simmer until agar flakes are dissolved. Pour juice into a shallow glass dish and refrigerate until set. Blend with tahini and spoon into individual parfait glasses. Garnish with cinnamon.

AYURVEDA DIET

Ayurveda originated in India over five thousand years ago and is still part of traditional Indian medicine. The word *Ayurveda* literally means "science of life." Until recently, Ayurveda was virtually unknown in the West; however, in the past few years, it has enjoyed notable interest throughout North America.

The underlying concept of Ayurveda is that health is natural and normal and everyone's birthright. Health is defined as the full functioning of digestion, assimilation, and elimination; a straight spine; and a harmony of body, mind, and spirit. Thus, health is not merely the absence of a definable disease, but rather a positive experience of well-being involving all aspects of an individual's life.

According to Ayurveda, human beings are composed of three fundamental mind/body principles, known as *doshas*. These three elements or doshas—*Vata, Pitta, Kapha*—govern all the psychological, physiological, and patho-physiological functions of mind and body. The specific proportion of the doshas (our basic nature) is determined at conception and generates each person's particular mental and physical style of functioning.

In addition to the original proportions of doshas, a person's dosha balance is influenced by each impulse of sensory experience that is processed by the nervous system. In other words, how we experience our day-to-day life events and relationships may alter our dosha balance and allow symptoms and illness to manifest.

We each possess all three doshas; however, one type or a combination of two types usually dominates within each of us. The three basic dosha types are described as follows.

ৡ VATA ৡ

Vata dosha governs all movement and activity, including mental, neuromuscular, circulatory, respiratory, and digestive functions. It is responsible for the circulation of information and nourishment throughout the body. A typical Vata constitution is light and thin in frame; has an active, restless, and creative mind; varies sleep and diet patterns; tolerates cold weather poorly; and may experience anxiety and insomnia when under stress.

❧ PITTA ❧

Pitta dosha governs metabolic and transformational functions. It is responsible for digestion, assimilation, body temperature, and the coloration of the skin, as well as strong emotions. A typical Pitta constitution has a moderate frame, a discriminating and keen intellect, a strong appetite and digestion, and warm extremities. Pittas perspire easily; and become irritable and angry under stress.

❧ KAPHA ❧

Kapha dosha maintains the structure of the body. It governs physical strength and stamina, joint lubrication, and respiratory tract secretions. A typical Kapha constitution has a heavyset build; a thoughtful, deliberate and methodical decision-making process; a slow, steady appetite and digestion; deep and prolonged sleep; and an easygoing, agreeable and balanced nature. Thus, Kaphas handle stress well.

From an ayurvedic perspective, to create and maintain good health it is essential to eat the right food at the right time in the appropriate manner and amounts. Food should be fresh and of the highest quality, and the diet should be chosen to suit the individual dosha constitution.

Ayurveda recognizes six major tastes/flavors in food which influence the doshas: sweet, salty, sour, pungent, bitter, and astringent. To insure satisfaction in eating, all six tastes should be present in each meal.

❧ *General guidelines for all doshas:*

- Eating should not be rushed, nor should it go on too long.
- Food should be:
    - warm or hot, therefore mostly cooked
    - tasty and easy to digest
    - eaten on an empty stomach and in the proper amount
    - eaten in a pleasant surrounding, utilizing the proper equipment

The following tridoshic menu has been carefully selected to fit the health needs of all dosha types.

ও AYURVEDA TRIDOSHIC MENU ও

Dahl Soup
Vegetable Curry served on Basmati Rice
Cucumber Raita
Date and Orange Chutney

Dahl Soup

1 tablespoon ghee (or butter)
1 small onion, minced
$^1/_2$ teaspoon cinnamon
$^1/_2$ teaspoon cumin
3 cups pink dahl beans or split mung beans
1 strip kombu seaweed
12 cups water
sea salt to taste
2 tablespoons fresh cilantro
lemon slices to garnish

ও *Serves 4–6*

In a heavy-bottomed saucepan, heat ghee and sauté onion with cinnamon and cumin until onion is limp and spices are fragrant. Add beans, kombu, and water; bring to a boil; cover, and simmer for 45 minutes to 1 hour. Salt to taste and garnish with chopped fresh cilantro and lemon slices.

Vegetable Curry

1 large butternut squash

2 tablespoons ghee

1 tablespoon curry

$1/2$ teaspoon cardamom

$1/2$ teaspoon cumin

$1/2$ teaspoon coriander

$1/2$ teaspoon ginger

$1/2$ teaspoon asafoetida (optional)

$1/2$ teaspoon anise seed

$1/2$ teaspoon turmeric

2 small onions, sliced

2 carrots, sliced diagonally

1 small cauliflower, cut into florets

1 cup green beans, cut into 2-inch strips

2 cups water

sea salt to taste

$1/3$ cup tahini

᠘ *Serves 4–6*

Cut butternut squash in half, remove seeds, and cut into pieces. (There's no need to peel it.) Place in a pot with water to almost cover, and boil until the pieces can be pierced with a fork. Purée in blender or food processor. Set aside.

In a heavy-bottomed saucepan, heat ghee and sauté spices with onion over medium/low flame, stirring frequently, until onion is limp and spices are fragrant. Add carrots, sauté a few minutes, add cauliflower, sauté a few more minutes, and then add beans. Add 2 cups cold water and sea salt to taste; cover, and simmer 15 minutes. Add tahini and puréed squash, stir, and heat throughly. Serve over Basmati rice.

Cucumber Raita

1 medium cucumber

1 cup nonfat yogurt

ঔ *Makes 1 cup*

Peel and seed cucumber, and finely chop. Combine with yogurt and serve with curried vegetables.

Date and Orange Chutney

1 whole orange, chopped

1 cup pitted dates, chopped

1 teaspoon fresh grated ginger

$1/3$ cup water

$1/3$ cup rice vinegar

1 tablespoon rice syrup

$1/4$ cup raisins

crushed chili pepper to taste

sea salt to taste

ঔ *Serves 4–6*

Combine all ingredients in a saucepan. Partially cover and cook over medium/low flame for 20–30 minutes. This chutney keeps well in the refrigerator for several weeks.

STARVING TO STUFFED

I'm gonna starve
if you don't take a bite
they tell me I'll get better
mileage on this machine
if I come clean.
Three days without food
I'm so used to baking
> *shopping*
> *stopping*
> *bopping*

for three squares
and now it appears
I'm still able to survive
on this reduced appetite.
Take a bite, less is more,
small is beautiful.
Honestly though, I wish for noodles
in which to dip my oodles.
Some starve on the face of our Earth.
Some choose to fast.
It's a way to be free I tell you
to be free of the past.
Take a rest, you'll be blest.
Oil change, rearrange DNA molecules, sharpen
your mind's eye
your heart
these are your tools. Open wide
make room inside for your song
and forever won't take long.
Time to get in tune
you don't want to be a ruin.
Free—enough for you, enough for me
the golden glee of the supersonic rainbonic key
sing it, sing it free.

—BETHANY S. ARGISLE

CHAPTER 10

DETOXIFICATION AND REJUVENATION

THE DIET TO CLEAN UP YOUR BODY, HEALTH AND LIFE

Our new cookbook just would not be complete without discussing the important process of detoxification and cleansing. I believe from both personal and medical practice experience that the cleansing process is crucial to long-term health in today's westernized cultures. In fact, I believe that fasting (cleansing) is the missing link in the American diet.

Illness occurs, nutritionally and biochemically, from two basic processes. The first is **deficiency**, whereby we are not getting enough of the essential nutrients we need. Deficiency may result from an imbalanced diet wherein certain foods are consumed in excess (at the exclusion of others) which do not provide basic vitamins, minerals, amino acids, and essential fatty acids. Deficiency may also occur in people with stressed and dysfunctioning digestive tracts, who then have reduced efficiency of assimilation.

People who are nutritionally deficient—and this could be experienced as fatigue and lack of endurance, coldness in the body, dry skin, hair loss, and other symptoms—need to eat good-quality, nutrient-rich foods on a regular basis. It is helpful to relax and chew food very well when eating, at least twenty to thirty times per mouthful.

Generally, most people in our culture have problems of **congestion**. Again these folks are getting an excess of certain substances and foods. Common congestive agents include refined flour and sugar products, breads and baked goods, fried foods and packaged foods made with hydrogenated fats, and excess animal proteins and fats, including cow's milk products. When all of this "stuff" cannot be utilized and eliminated daily, it clogs our cells and tissues and leads to poor internal respiration and poor function on a cellular level. This internal congestion leads to blocked sinuses, skin eruptions and rashes, muscular aches and pains, allergy symptoms, headaches, and more.

Certain biochemical conditions in the body cause increased toxicity, and the body increases its accumulation of wastes and elimination in order to maintain its deeper level of health. Therefore, in a naturopathic understanding, the body's symptoms are its attempt to preserve health or make itself better. This toxicity state is one of excess acid and mucus, and the eliminative by-products are the same.

Commonly, the people accumulating excesses are also not acquiring all of their necessary nutrients; thus, they may simultaneously have problems of congestion and deficiency. It follows that by detoxifying with certain foods, such people can also be nourished—cleansed at the same time they are receiving the very nutrients they lack. The Alkaline Detoxification Diet is ideal for such needs.

The eating plan for this diet usually lasts several weeks, and primarily includes foods that create an alkaline residue when utilized in our bodies. This allows the acid congestions in the body to be balanced and released, and mucus waste products to be eliminated through the normal channels. We discussed acid-alkaline balance in Chapter 1 of this book, where we concluded that for long-term health, our diets should abound with more alkaline-forming foods—fruits and vegetables, whole grains (especially millet and buckwheat), and almonds and bean sprouts for protein. These foods should constitute two-thirds of our diet, and ideally the fruit and vegetable components should be half of our entire daily consumption.

Literally thousands of my patients over recent years have followed the Alkaline Detoxification Diet, and I have used it myself twice for about one month each time. In *Staying Healthy with Nutrition*, I thoroughly discuss the detoxification process and practice. Many readers and reviewers feel that this section of the book is the most extensive and up-to-date discussion on detoxification in print. This diet was tested and written up in the January/February 1993 issue of *Natural Health* magazine. People feel good on this diet and many of their congestive symptoms are eliminated. However, if they go back on their congestive diets, their symptoms often return.

The Alkaline Detoxification Diet gives the body a more alkaline biochemistry, and allows the easier elimination or balancing of protein and acid wastes that create inflammatory and degenerative changes in the body. As I mentioned earlier, much of the congestive acid and mucus wastes come from the use of refined foods and protein/fat foods, especially the overuse of animal products. Reducing these foods for life and specifically with this detox diet will begin the positive shifts necessary for improved health.

This detoxification diet is a key to healing. After three to four weeks, we can assess, if we pay attention, how what we do and what we eat affects our state of health and symptoms. Subsequently, we can learn what to avoid to maintain this healthier, cleaner, more energetic, and less symptomatic state.

THE ALKALINE DETOXIFICATION DIET

3–4 WEEK PROGRAM

This diet focuses on chewing well (twenty to thirty times per mouthful), eating mostly vegetables, drinking quality water and the water from steamed vegetables, and eating all food prior to nightfall, advisedly before 6:30 P.M. Here are the guidelines for the diet:

1. Chew very well and take your time when you eat.

2. Relax a few minutes before and after your meal.

3. Eat in a comfortable sitting position.

4. Eat primarily steamed fresh vegetables and some fresh greens.

5. Take only herbal teas after dinner.

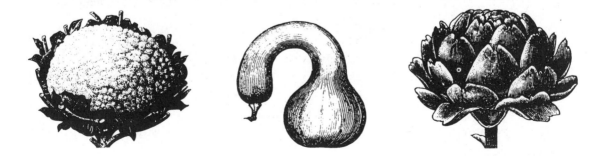

❧ THE ALKALINE-DETOXIFICATION MENU PLAN ❧

Morning: (**upon rising**) Two glasses of water (filtered or spring), one glass with half a lemon squeezed into it.

Breakfast: One piece of fresh fruit (at room temperature), such as an apple, pear, banana, a citrus fruit, or some grapes. Chew well, mixing each bite with saliva.

Fifteen to thirty minutes later: One bowl of cooked whole grains—specifically millet, brown rice, amaranth, quinoa, or buckwheat.

For flavoring use two tablespoons of fruit juice for sweetness, or use the Better Butter mixture mentioned below with a little salt or tamari for a savory taste.

Lunch: (Noon-1 P.M.) One to two medium bowls of steamed vegetables; use a variety, including roots, stems, and greens. For example, potatoes or yams, green beans, broccoli or cauliflower, carrots or beets, asparagus, kale, chard, and cabbage. Be sure to *chew well!*

Dinner: (5-6 P.M.): Same as lunch.

Seasoning: butter/canola oil (cold-pressed) mixture. Make *Better Butter* by mixing a quarter-cup of cold-pressed canola oil into a soft (room temperature) quarter-pound of butter; then place in dish and refrigerate. Use about one teaspoon per meal or a maximum of 3 teaspoons daily.

11 A.M. & 3 P.M. One to two cups veggie water, saved from the steamed vegetables. Add a little sea salt or kelp and drink slowly, mixing each mouthful with saliva.

Evening: Herbal teas, such as peppermint, camomile, pau d'arco, or blends.

NOTE: You may feel a little weak or have symptoms such as fatigue, headaches, or irritability for the first couple of days; these will pass. A feeling of clarity should appear by the third or fourth day, if not sooner. If during this diet you start to feel weak or hungry, assess your water intake and elimination; if needed, you can eat a small portion of protein food (three to four ounces) in the mid-afternoon. This could be fish; free-range, organic chicken; or some beans, such as lentils, garbanzos, mung, or black beans.

SEASONAL SUGGESTIONS FOR DETOXIFICATION VEGETABLES

Try steaming basic combinations that include some root vegetables, tubers, stems, leafy greens, and vegetable fruits (from flowering vines that give such veggies as zucchini, green beans, and peppers).

Spring	• Asparagus, baby carrots, spring garlic, red chard • Beets, leeks, broccoli, wild greens such as mustard, sorrel or collard, with a steamed artichoke
Summer	• Zucchini, new potatoes, green beans, carrots, onion • Beets and beet greens, yellow squash, bell pepper, eggplant
Autumn	• Broccoli, cabbage, potato, celery, spinach • Cauliflower, onion, carrots, chard, sugar peas
Winter	• Broccoli, cabbage, potato, kale, spinach, chard • Butternut squash, onion, cauliflower, collard greens, Jerusalem artichoke
Seasonings	• A little bit of sea salt, vegetable salt, or a good garlic salt without additives can be used; cayenne adds warmth. • *Better Butter* (see recipe p. 234) is a must for the Alkaline Detoxification Diet, preventing deficiencies of essential fatty acids (see Fat-Free Diets discussion on p. 211). The mixture of butter and cold-pressed canola oil provides all the fatty acids to nourish and support the tissues.

❧ FASTING ❧

For more advanced health concerns, certain long-term illnesses, excess weight, or when the need for a stronger transformation is present, a juice cleanse may be useful. I am a believer in the fasting process; however, this process is best used as a transition to an improved diet and eating habits, not as a weight-loss program. During autumn and winter I tend to become congested easily and gain a few pounds; during spring and summer I may have allergy symptoms. I find that the cleansing process of a juice fast is a perfect healing and rebalancing tool for me. I have done a ten-day juice fast every spring for the last nineteen years; it always revitalizes me and prepares me for a healthier, lighter diet in the warmer months. The Master Cleanser Diet is what I usually do, and most often I drag along another twenty to thirty patients and friends to do it with me for support, and although it is not always an easy ride, almost all are thrilled by the experience.

The Master Cleanser formula is: 2 tablespoons of fresh squeezed lemon or lime juice; 1–2 tablespoons of pure, 100% maple syrup; and $1/10$ teaspoon cayenne pepper, all mixed in eight ounces of water, preferably pure spring water. You can adjust this slightly to your taste, but most people find this a good balance of flavors—sweet, sour, and spicy.

Lemon is a perfect liver food and a great body cleanser. High in vitamin C, potassium, and other minerals, lemons are somewhat astringent. They contract and tighten tissues, loosening the toxins from deep tissues and organs. The cayenne pepper helps clear the blood, eliminate toxins and mucus, and keep the body warm. The maple syrup is wonderful energy (calories, too), and it, along with honey, is a primary natural sugar. You may vary the calories and sweetness by using less maple syrup, depending on the weight loss you desire—which can be up to two pounds a day, especially with lots of activity. Honey is not acceptable in this drink, as it is congesting in amounts needed.

Drink Master Cleanser throughout the day, at least six glasses a day. One to two weeks is not too difficult or too long for this cleanse.

I have written about fasting in both of the *Staying Healthy* books. I refer you to the Spring section of *Staying Healthy with the Seasons* and to Chapter 18 of *Staying Healthy with Nutrition* for more extensive discussions and additional guidelines on cleansing the body.

After two decades of working with thousands of fasting and detoxing patients, I can say to you that cleansing the body is a powerful healing process that frees the spirit and helps you align (or re-align) your life by enhancing your overall health.

CHAPTER 11
OTHER HEALTH GUIDELINES

I want here to succintly address some important basic guidelines, beyond nutrition, for your healthy living and long life. Please remember that your health and how you feel is an outcome of your life to date—your genetics and constitution, your upbringing and childhood support system (which influences your attitudes, disposition and your approach to life), your past health problems and how you treated them, your diet and exercise patterns, your stress level, your challenges, your work and the satisfaction you take in it, your personal relationships, and, your emotional health and support. All of these elements contribute to your well-being as well as to your health. Symptoms and illness itself are exacerbated, if not caused, by such factors in your life. Being able to sense this and make appropriate changes is the beginning of your real healing process.

There are four cornerstones of good health and preventive medicine: **nutrition, exercise, attitude,** and **stress management**. Nutrition and exercise go hand-in-hand to create health; one without the other does not work as well. Your basic exercise plan should be simple and balanced, as well as consistent. Your regular program must include stretching to enhance flexibility, aerobic activity to gain endurance, and some weight training to build strength and tone. This regular, balanced plan will improve your relaxation and coordination and give you abundant energy. If you desire long-term weight control, good health, and vitality, you must exercise regularly and safely. Seek out the appropriate instructors or books to help you in setting up the best plan for you, and then make it a part of your life three to five times per week.

The other two building blocks of good health are attitude and stress management.

Your attitude influences how you care for yourself—whether you create and accept regular abuse nutritionally and emotionally, or whether you live a health-enhancing lifestyle. Finding playful and relaxing activities to balance out stress is also essential for health maintenance. Learning to take a less aggressive, more open approach to life is important.

Often, the first level that I look at in an individual's health improvement plan is their regular use and abuse of mind or energy-altering substances, such as caffeine, alcohol, nicotine, or sugar. (Specific detoxification programs for caffeine, alcohol, nicotine, and other drugs are fully discussed in Chapter 18 of *Staying Healthy with Nutrition*.) Even refined carbohydrates, like bread and baked goods, may offer emotional (not always nutritional) support for some people. Healing abuses and addictions is a crucial component of good nutrition and lifelong health; therefore, it is imperative to create a plan for changing these often long-term destructive habits, which all stem from learned behavior patterns for coping emotionally with life events and traumas.

Here are some guidelines for healing abuses and addictions:

* Address underlying emotions

* Gather willpower

* Create a plan

* Use the Detoxification Diet to alkalinize the body (see Chapter 10)

* Drink water

* Exercise regularly

* Take vitamins, such as vitamin C, the B vitamins, and extra antioxidants (beta-carotene, vitamin E and selenium; see pp. 35–37)

* Take minerals, like calcium, magnesium, and chromium (see pp. 35–37)

Another health guideline: drink water as the primary liquid in your diet. Avoid the regular use of soda, coffee, and black tea, and even excessive bottled juices. Regular water intake helps to maintain body balance, proper internal organ function (especially of the digestive tract) and proper elimination. It is also an important component for weight control and long-term weight management. Eight glasses a day is a basic recommendation, and this may vary depending on a number of factors. These factors are discussed in detail in Chapter 1 of *Staying Healthy with Nutrition*, along with which type of water is the best quality and least toxic: namely, water filtered through a solid carbon block or a reverse osmosis unit. It is best to drink water away from meals: two to three glasses to start the day, and then a glass or two about thirty minutes to an hour before a meal to reduce cravings and the desire to overeat. When working with weight control, programming yourself to drink a glass or two of water instead of putting that snack in your mouth is a healthy habit to develop.

I call my approach to medicine *integrated,* not *holistic* or *alternative*. Integrated Medicine utilizes many modalities and ideally designs the simplest, safest, and most efficacious treatment for a given health situation. As a conscientious consumer, it is wise to develop knowledge about over-the-counter nutritional supplements available to you such as vitamins, minerals, herbs, and homeopathic remedies.

There are four levels of Integrated Medicine which I consider fundamental. First is the integration of preventive care with family practice diagnosis and treatment. Traditional Western medicine is often greatly enhanced by natural remedies, counseling, acupuncture, and body work, for example.

Next, there is the blending of multidisciplinary practices—conventional medicine with more natural methods. These include using pharmaceutical *and* nutritional/herbal supplements (with a physician's guidance); osteopathic care along with other physical therapies; and stress management with general lifestyle guidance.

The third aspect of Integrated Medicine relates to addressing different levels of the human being—physical, mental, emotional, and spiritual. Herein lies the foundation of what has been termed "holistic medicine." Integrated Medicine looks at an individual's whole life rather than focusing solely on physical symptoms, and then uses this information for evaluation and treatment.

The final and possibly the most important factor involves moving away from the "fix-it" model of Western medicine into the integrative practice of understanding health as an outcome of one's life. How you live, think, act; what you eat and how you digest; your level of stress and attitude toward life; your genetics and upbringing; your past problems and how you dealt with them—all of these and more contribute to the person you are and the state you are in. If you want this person, this you, to be different, then you need to pay attention to the factors in your life that are contributing to your current health or illness, and support or change them. Take special care to notice the outcome of these changes. A new lifestyle creates a new body, a shift in energy, and will undoubtedly create many other positive effects in your life.

In most healing processes, I find that people need to become more aware, more sensitive to subtler aspects of both their outer and inner lives—particularly emotional and psychological issues. Acupuncture and certain types of bodywork deal with subtle levels of energy to stimulate a deeper awareness. From here, issues can be dealt with more presently and cleared from the body/mind, where they have created an imbalanced state.

One way to accomplish deeper healing is to find a process that can generate insight and understanding, leading to inner transformation. The real shift comes from how you approach your ill health, both in attitude and in practice. Looking at illness as a positive force for change is useful. Moving from the question, "What should I take to make this go away?" to potentially more important questions, like "Why is this problem or symptom happening?", "Body, what are you trying to tell me?", and "What do I need to do to really heal?" will begin the new process of mending the separation that happens at the different levels of your being when you ignore your body. Taking an integrated approach to health is the first step to health empowerment and *becoming your own best doctor*. Eating well and following the simple, natural, seasonal, and wholesome approach laid out in this book is the beginning of that transformation.

Good Luck and Bon Appétit!

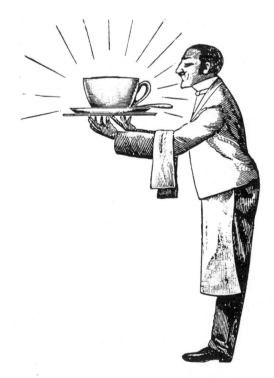

NUTRITIONAL ANALYSIS OF THE SEASONAL DIETS

	RDA	Spring	Summer	Autumn	Winter
Constituents					
Calories	1,300–2,000	1,500	1,500	1,650	1,880
Carbohydrates (g)	200	190	180	200	225
Cholesterol (mg)	under 300	100	160	105	130
Fats (g)	25–75	55	48	54	65
Protein (g)	56	60	65	70	76
Fiber (g)	NE*(10)	10	10	12	15
Water (liter)	2.5	2.6	2.9	2.7	2.8
Vitamins					
Vitamin A/Beta-Carotene (IU)	5,000	14,000	14,000	18,000	22,000
Thiamine (B1) (mg)	1.4	1.5	1.3	1.4	1.7
Riboflavin (B2) (mg)	1.6	1.6	1.4	1.6	1.8
Niacin (B3) (mg)	18	20	19	18	24
Pantothenic Acid (B5) (mg)	5	6	6	9	11
Pyridoxine (B6) (mg)	2	3	3	2.6	3.4
Cobalamin (B12) (mcg)	3	0.6	1.0	0.6	1.3
Folic Acid (mcg)	400	450	400	460	480
Vitamin C (mg)	45	175	200	180	240
Vitamin E (IU)	15	14	10	12	15
Vitamin K (mcg)	300	340	240	500	320
Minerals					
Calcium (Ca) (mg)	800	500	640	490	800
Copper (Cu) (mg)	2.0	3.1	7	3.4	38
Iron (Fe) (mg)	10–18	16	18	16	18
Magnesium (Mg) (mg)	350	340	340	360	440
Potassium (K) (mg)	2.5	3.2	3.1	3.5	4.4
Phosphorus (P) (mg)	800	1,150	1,200	1,100	1,400
Sodium (Na) (mg)	2	1.4	1.5	1.4	2.4
Zinc (Zn) (mg)	15	12	20	13	16

* NE — Not established.

NOTE: Values, of course, will vary with the quality and amount of food consumed. The seasonal diets, mostly vegetarian and low fat, reveal slightly low values for certain nutrients in these analyses. Vitamins and minerals to watch include most of the B vitamins, especially B12, calcium, zinc, and iron for women. These diets are very high in Vitamin A and potassium levels, and low in cholesterol and sodium. You can do an analysis of your diet using a book that includes food values or with a practitioner who uses a special nutritional service.

RECIPE BOOK BIBLIOGRAPHY

Airola Diet and Cookbook, Paavo Airola (Phoenix, AZ: Health Plus Publishers, 1981). Paavo Airola provides some very simple and vital recipes; a good overall program for lighter eating. This book can be ordered directly from the publisher by writing to Health Plus Publishers, P.O. Box 22001, Phoenix, AZ 85028.

Book of Whole Meals: A Seasonal Guide to Assembling Balanced Vegetarian Breakfasts, Lunches, and Dinners, Annemarie Colbin (New York, NY: Ballantine Books, 1985). Annemarie Colbin includes many fine yet simple recipes in this macrobiotic-oriented book. This book can be obtained directly from the publisher by calling (800)733-3000. Her newest publication is *The Natural Gourmet*.

Cosmic Cookery, out of print, Kathryn Hannaford (Stockton, CA: Starmast Publications, 1974).

Dr. Braly's Food Allergy and Nutrition Revolution, James Braly (New Canaan, CT: Keats Publishing, Inc., 1992). A reprint of *Dr. Braly's Optimum Health Program,* this book offers a current perspective on food allergies and illness.

Eat Well, Be Well Cookbook, Metropolitan Life Insurance Co. (New York, NY: Fireside, 1986). A lower-fat, "heart-healthy" version of an American diet; includes some use of sugar and chemicals, but has many interesting recipes.

Enchanted Broccoli Forest (Revised), Mollie Katzen (Berkeley, CA: Ten Speed Press, 1982, 1995).

Fast Vegetarian Feasts, rev. ed., Martha Rose Shulman (New York, NY: Dolphin Books, 1986). One of the best cookbooks I've seen: well-organized, good recipes from basic natural ingredients, low fat, and even a seasonal orientation. Love it!

Fit for Life, Harvey Diamond and Marilyn Diamond (New York, NY: Warner Books, 1987). Although the authors' focus is food philosophy, they provide a number of simple, wholesome, and tasty recipes.

Moosewood Cookbook (Revised), Mollie Katzen (Berkeley, CA: Ten Speed Press, 1992).

Hippocrates Diet and Health Program, Ann Wigmore (Garden City Park, NY: Avery Publishing Group, 1984). A unique book for the diet-conscious who enjoy sprouts and raw foods. Purifying, vital, and extremely healthy.

New Laurel's Kitchen, 2nd ed., Laurel Robertson, Carol Flinders, and Brian Ruppenthal (Berkeley, CA: Ten Speed Press, 1986). Very popular, well-rounded, and good for the basics. The original version was too heavy in milk products and sugar for optimum health; the new version published by Ten Speed Press is much improved.

Self-Healing Cookbook: A Macrobiotic Primer for Healing Body, Mind and Moods with Whole, Natural Foods, 2nd, rev. ed., Kristina Turner (Grass Valley, CA: Earthtones Press, 1988). A very healthful, practical, and easy-to-use recipe book.

Still Life With Menu Cookbook (Revised), Mollie Katzen (Berkeley, CA: Ten Speed Press, 1994). A beautiful and elegant book with some wonderful recipes. Mollie Katzen's newest cookbook follows her popular *Moosewood Cookbook (Revised)* and *Enchanted Broccoli Forest (Revised)*.

Stress, Diet, and Your Heart, Dean Ornish, MD (New York, NY: New American Library, 1984). Dr. Dean Ornish wrote this winning book with many healthful, creative recipes; a special book for heart patients. Look for his new book, *Dr. Dean Ornish's Program for Reversing Heart Disease*.

The Tao of Cooking, Sally Pasley (Berkeley, CA: Ten Speed Press, 1982). Popular for many years, this nicely balanced book includes many simple, tasty recipes.

Tropic Cooking, Joyce Lefray Young (Berkeley, CA: Ten Speed Press, 1987). Delectable and nutritionally-balanced recipes make up this book, filled with exotic recipes from Florida to the Caribbean Islands.

INDEX

A

Abuses, healing, 238
Acid-alkaline balance, 21
Acid-alkaline foods, 21, 29
Addictions, healing, 238
Additives, in American diet, 22
Airola, Paavo, 67, 108, 162
Alkaline detoxification
    diet, 232-35
    menu plan, 234
Allergy, 85
    causes, 13
Almonds, toasted, 60
Amino acids, list, 18
Apple
    baked, 193
    mousse, 224
    pie, 219
Apple-raisin compote, 181
Apricot
    bars, 139
    and prune compote, 146

ArgIsle, Bethany, 202
Artichoke stew, 101
Aspic, tofu, 126
Attitude, 1, 237
Autumn foods list, 172
Avocado dressing, 90
Ayurveda diet, 210, 225-29

B

Balance
    acid-alkaline, 21
    aspects, 16
    color, 19-20
    diet, 16-21
    flavor, 19-20
    food groups, 19
    macronutrients, 16-17
    micronutrients, 17-18
Barley, cooking, 40
Bass with pepper sauce, 159
Bean
    and cabbage soup, 194
    dip, 70
    purée, 212

    soup, 100
    spread, 70
    stew, 181
Beans,
    cooking times, 41
    reducing gas from,
      41, 44
    seasoning, 42
    use of salt, 41
    washing, 41
Beet salad, 131
Bok choy, 224
Borscht, 195
Braley, James, 65, 201
Bread
    carrot, 169
    pudding, 215
Broccoli soup, 176
Brody, Jane, 22
Broth, vegetable, 54
Brown, Edward Espe, 243
Brownies, carob, 203
Bulgur substitute, 165
Burgers, vegetable, 164

Butter
  carrot, 71
  onion-miso, 46
  peanut-apple, 123
  squash, 72

C

Cabbage
  kasha stuffed, 199
  sweet & sour, 168
Cake
  millet, 148
  quinoa, 75
Candy, tahini, 79
Carbohydrates sources, 17
Cardiovascular disease diet, 209
Carrot
  butter, 71
  bread, 169
  hash browns, 170
  soup, 91
Cauliflower and
  bechamel sauce, 191
Chard, stuffed, 128
Cheese, seed, 69
Chicken
  baked in paper, 120
  curried, 180
  sautéed, 157
Chili, vegetarian, 200
Chop Suey, 60
Chopra, Deepak, 210
Chronic disease, 23
  and fats, 211

Chutney, 229
Cleaning
  dressing for, 108
  vegetables, 40-42
Colbin, Annemarie, 39-40, 79, 109, 161
Coleslaw, 129
Color, versus body function, 20
Congestion, 231-32
Cookies
  almond, 81
  apricot bars, 139
  carob brownies, 203
  fruit bars, 80
  oatmeal, 179
Cooking methods, macrobiotic, 221
Corn
  gaspacho, 217
  stew, 183
  and tomato soup, 130
Corn bread, 123
  jalapeño, 167
Couscous, 136
  flan, 214
  salad, 95
Cracked wheat, 176
Crackers, 65
Crepes, 118
Croquettes, millet, 150
Cucumber raita, 229
Curry
  chicken, 180
  vegetable, 102, 228

D

Dahl soup, 227
Deficiency, nutritional, 231
Dessert
  apple-raisin compote, 181
  baked apple, 193
  cakes, 75, 148
  frozen, 138
  jelled fruit, 121
  nice cream, 77
  pears, 155
  pies, 185, 204, 219
  puddings, 99, 215
  pumpkin pie, 185
Detoxification, 231-36
  diet, 141, 209
  vegetables for, 235
Detoxifiers, 87
Diamond, Harvey, 170
Diamond, Marilyn, 170
Diet
  alkaline detoxification, 232-35
  Ayurveda, 210, 225-29
  balance, 16-21
  cardiovascular, 209
  characteristics of ideal, 30
  components of healthy, 10
  definition of ideal, 25
  detoxification, 141, 209
  fat-free, 209, 211-15
  4-day rotation, 85
  guidelines for healthy, 7
  guidelines for ideal, 26
  ideal, 1, 25-27

indigenous, 11
macrobiotic, 209, 220-24
master cleanser, 235-36
natural hygiene, 209, 216-19
nutritional analysis of seasonal, 241
omnivore, 26
pescovegan, 86
purpose of ideal, 27
raw-foods, 68, 209, 216-19
rotation, 13-14
sample of ideal, 31
schedule for ideal, 32-34
seasonal, 1
statistics on daily, 34
supplements, 35-37
variety, 13
vegan, 26
vegetarian, 26
Dip, bean, 70
Doshas, 225-26
Dressing
avocado, 90
hot & sour, 197
miso, 53
miso-tahini, 92
parsley, 109
pollution solution, 108
raspberry yogurt, 74
tao, 133

E

Eating advice, 3
Endive salad, 125
Essential nutrients, 18
Exercise, 1, 237

F

Fasting, 87, 231, 235-36
Fat-free diet, 209, 211-15
Fats
and chronic disease, 211
sources, 17
substitute, 45-46
Feijoada, 151
Fettuccine and curried vegetables, 102
Fish
bass, 159
buying tips, 43
salmon, 125
snapper, 182
sole, 144
swordfish, 152
Flan, couscous, 214
Flatulence
cause, 221
reducing, 41, 44
Flinders, Carol, 61, 130, 139, 165-66
Food groups
balance, 19
new, 3, 9
old, 8-9
omnivorous, 19
vegetarian, 19
Foods
acid-alkaline, 21, 29
bad combinations, 14
chemically clean, 12
combining, 14-15
good combinations, 15
list of autumn, 172
list of spring, 111
list of summer, 140

list of winter, 205
natural benefits, 11
natural flavor, 13
organic, 12
seasonal, 11
storage, 46
French fries, substitute, 164
Frozen fruit desserts, 77
Frozen juice pops, 76
Frozen yogurt desserts, 77, 138
Fruit
bars, 80, 139
compote, 146
jelled in dessert, 121

G

Garlic
soup, 162
sauce, 215
Thai soup, 163
Gaspacho, corn, 217
Gomasio, 58
Grain
cooking times, 40
washing, 39
Granola, 48
Gravy thickeners, 45
Guacamole, 56

H

Halvah, 79
Hannaford, Kathryn, 169, 203
Health Bank Account, 2
Health guidelines

Health Guidelines *con't*
  diet, 7, 26
  non-nutritional, 237-40
Hot & sour
  dressing, 197
  soup, 196
Hummus, 218

I

Icing, carob, 203
Ideal diet, 1, 25-27
  characteristics, 30
  definition, 25
  guidelines, 26
  purpose, 27
  sample, 31
  schedule, 32-34
Indigenous diet, 11
Integrated medicine, 239

J

'Jello', natural, 121
Juice pops, 76

K

Kanten, fruit, 121
Kapha, 226
Kasha
  cooking, 40
  cream, 161
  definition, 161
  stuffing, 198
Katzen, Mollie, 63, 67, 110,
  131-32, 137, 163, 195,
  200
Kelley, William Donald, 27

Ketchup, 61
Kitchen shortcuts, 44
Kushi, Aveline, 220
Kushi, Michio, 220

L

Lasagna, 145
Leeks and bechamel sauce,
  191
Lemon sauce, 75
Lentil soup, 184

M

Macaroni and tofu au
  gratin, 192
Macrobiotic
  cooking methods, 221
  diet, 209, 220-24
Macronutrients, 16-17
  sources, 17
Marination, quick, 45
Master cleanser
  diet, 235-36
  fast, 87
  formula, 236
Mayonnaise
  ethnic, 67
  tofu, 67
McDougall, John, 209
Menu plans
  alkaline detoxification,
    234
  autumn, 142
  spring, 88-89
  summer, 114
  winter, 174-75

Metabolic types, 27-29
  parasympathetic, 28
  sympathetic, 28
Metal poisoning, 108
Micronutrients, 17-18
Milk
  nut, 78
  substitute, 46
Millet
  cake, 148
  cooking, 40
  croquettes, 150
  substitute, 165
Minerals list, 18
Minestrone, 93
Miso dressing, 53
Miso-tahini dressing, 92
Moussaka, 122
Mousse
  apple, 224
  carob-tofu, 147
Mushroom
  sauce, 177
  soup, 222

N

Natural foods, benefits, 10
Natural hygiene diet, 209,
  216-19
Nice cream, 77
Nut milk, 78
Nut sauce, 201
Nutrients, essential, 18
Nutritional analysis,
  seasonal diets, 241

Nutritional deficiency, 231

Nuts, storage, 11

O

Oatmeal cookies, 179

Obesity, causes, 15-16

Ohsawa, George, 220

Oils, flavored, 45

Omnivore, diet, 26

Omnivorous, food groups, 19

Onion soup, 190

Onion-miso butter, 46

Orange sauce, 148

Organic foods, 12

Ornish, Dean, 52, 197, 204, 209

P

Peanut-apple butter, 123

Parasympathetic metabolic type, 28

Pasley, Sally, 106, 133-34

Pasta
    and beans, 90
    and curried vegetables, 102
    and greens, 110
    mushroom, 154
    with vegetables, 137

Pea soup, 160

Pears, 155

Peeling
    tomato, 136
    vegetables, 42

Pepper coulis, 159

Peppers, stuffed bell, 117

Pescovegan diet, 86

Pesto sauce, 94

Pie
    banana cream, 204
    pumpkin, 185
    raw apple, 219
    wheat-free crust, 64

Pitta, 226

Pizza
    instant, 45
    rice crust, 135

Polenta, 96

Potato casserole, 156

Potatoes
    mashed, 158
    natural French 'fries', 76

Pressure cooker, precautions, 40-41

Proteins, sources, 17

Prune and apricot compote, 146

Pudding
    bread, 215
    strawberry-rhubarb, 99

Pumpkin pie, 185

Q

Quinoa
    cake, 75
    cooking, 40
    and peppers, 165
    salad, 74
    and spinach, 73

R

Raita, cucumber, 229

Raspberry dressing, 74

Ratatouille, 127

Raw-foods diet, 68, 209, 216-19

RDA, Recommended Daily Allowance
    mineral, 37, 241
    vitamin, 36, 241

Red cabbage salad, 153

Rejuvelac, 68-69

Rice
    balls, 80
    and beans, 103, 223
    breakfast, 116
    cooking brown, 39
    and eggs, 202
    and lentil loaf, 188
    salad, 51, 109
    and vegetables, 59

Robertson, Laurel, 61, 130, 139, 165-66

Ruppenthal, Brian, 61, 130, 139, 165-66

S

SAD. *See* Standard American diet

Salad
    beet, 131
    couscous, 95
    endive, 125
    general ingredients, 49
    Mexican, 124
    mixed sprout, 50
    quinoa, 74

Salad *con't*
   red cabbage, 153
   rice, 51, 109
   spinach, 150
   tao, 133
   vegetable, 132
   watercress, 107
Salmon, baked, 125
Salsa, 56
Salt
   benefits of sea, 43
   sesame, 58
Sauce
   creamy tofu, 199
   garlic, 215
   green, 189
   Italian, 62
   lemon, 75
   Mexican, 62
   mushroom, 177
   nut, 201
   orange, 148
   parsley-mint, 214
   pesto, 94
   sweet & sour, 98
   tomato, 62-63
   tomato-caper, 92
   tomato-lentil, 96
   walnut-miso, 147
Sauerkraut, 218
Seasonal diet, 1
Seasonal foods, 11
Seasoning
   beans, 42
   ethnic, 43
   general mixture, 44
   removing excess, 43
Seed cheese, 69

Seed yogurt, 69
Seeds, storage, 11
Sesame salt, 58
Shortcuts, kitchen, 44
Shoyu, definition, 187
Shrimp, 105
Shrimp Creole, 171
Shulman, Martha Rose, 138, 167-68, 196, 198-99
Snapper, parmentière, 182
Sodium, substitute, 45
Sole, baked, 144
Sorbet, 121
Soup
   bean and cabbage, 194
   carrot, 91
   Chinese vegetable, 106
   corn & tomato, 130
   cream of broccoli, 176
   cream of garlic, 162
   dahl, 227
   garlic, 162
   hot & sour, 196
   lentil, 184
   mushroom miso, 222
   onion, 190
   split pea, 160
   Thai garlic, 163
   vegetable, 54-55
   vegetable cream, 55
   white bean, 100
Sour cream
   substitute, 46
   tofu, 66
Spinach
   and quinoa, 73
   salad, 150

Spread
   bean, 70
   butter-free, 71-72
   carrot, 71
   squash, 72
   tofu nut, 81
Spring foods list, 111
Squash bisque, 186
Squash butter, 72
Standard American diet, 22
   problems, 22
Stew
   artichoke, 101
   bean, 181
   corn, 183
Storage
   food, 46
   nuts and seeds, 11
Strawberry-rhubarb pudding, 99
Stress management, 1, 237
Stuffing, kasha, 198
Substitute
   bulgur, 165
   fat, 45-46
   French fries, 164
   milk, 46
   millet, 165
   sodium, 45
   sour cream, 46
   for stir-frying, 46
Summer foods list, 140
Sushi, 187
Sweet & sour cabbage, 168
Sweet & sour sauce, 98
Sweet & sour tofu, 98
Sweet & sour tempeh, 98

Swordfish, broiled, 152

Sympathetic metabolic type, 28

T

Tahini candy, 79

Tempeh
  cacciatore, 166
  sweet & sour, 98
  and vegetables, 178

Tofu
  aspic, 126
  banana cream pie, 204
  and carob mousse, 147
  creamy sauce, 199
  mayonnaise, 67
  nut spread, 81
  scrambled, 119
  sour cream, 66
  sweet & sour, 98
  topping, 146
  and vegetables, 178
  zucchini stuffing, 104

Tofunaise, 91

Tomato
  and corn soup, 130
  peeling, 136
  sauce, 62
  vinaigrette, 213

Tomato-caper sauce, 92

Tomato-lentil sauce, 96

Topping, tofu, 146

Tostadas, 57

Turkey
  baked, 149
  roasted, 177

Turner, Kristina, 64, 71, 149

V

Vata, 225

Vegan diet, 26. *See also*
  Natural hygiene diet;
  Pescovegan

Vegetable
  broth, 54
  burger, 164
  chili, 200
  cream soup, 55
  curry, 228
  salad, 132
  soup, 54-55

Vegetables
  and pasta, 137
  and rice, 59
  for detoxification, 42
    235
  peeling, 42
  steamed, 58
  and tempeh, 178
  and tofu, 178
  windowpane cut, 178

Vegetarian
  Ayurveda diet, 210
  chili, 200
  diet, 26
  food groups, 19

Vinaigrette
  honey mustard, 122
  low salt & fat, 52
  tomato, 213

Vitamin list, 18

W

Walnut-miso sauce, 147

Wasabi, definition, 187

Water in the diet, 238-39

Watercress
  bisque, 97
  salad, 107

Wheat, cracked, 176

Wigmore, Ann, 68

Windowpane cut, 178

Winter foods list, 205

Y

Yogurt freezes, 77

Yogurt, seed, 69

Young, Joyce LeFray, 105

Z

Zucchini, 134
  stuffed flowers, 104